The Science of Play

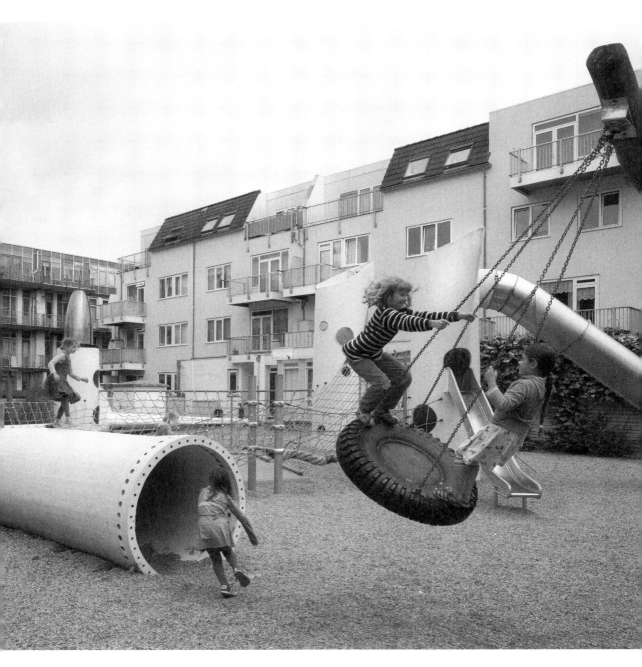

The Science of

University Press of New England

Hanover and London

SUSAN G. SOLOMON

PLAY

How to Build Playgrounds That Enhance
Children's Development

University Press of New England
www.upne.com
© 2014 University Press of New England
All rights reserved
Manufactured in the United States of America
Designed by Eric M. Brooks
Typeset in Calluna by Passumpsic Publishing

For permission to reproduce any of the material in this
book, contact Permissions, University Press of New England,
One Court Street, Suite 250, Lebanon NH 03766;
or visit www.upne.com

Library of Congress Cataloging-in-Publication Data
available upon request

5 4 3 2 1

for Bob

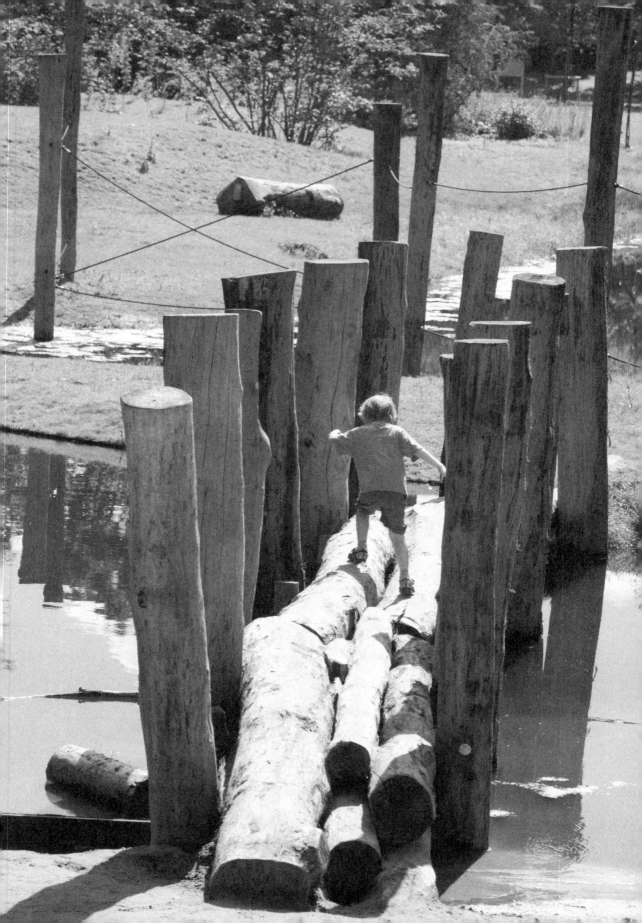

Life demands courage, endurance and strength,

but we continue to underestimate the capacity of children

for taking risks, enjoying the stimulation of danger,

and finding things out for themselves.

LADY ALLEN OF HURTWOOD

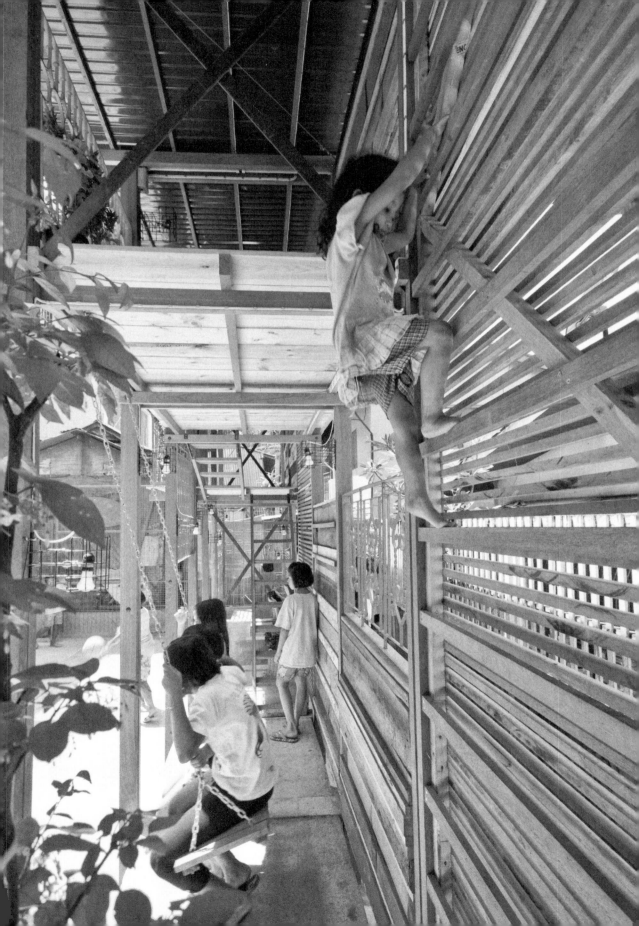

Contents

Plates follow page 82

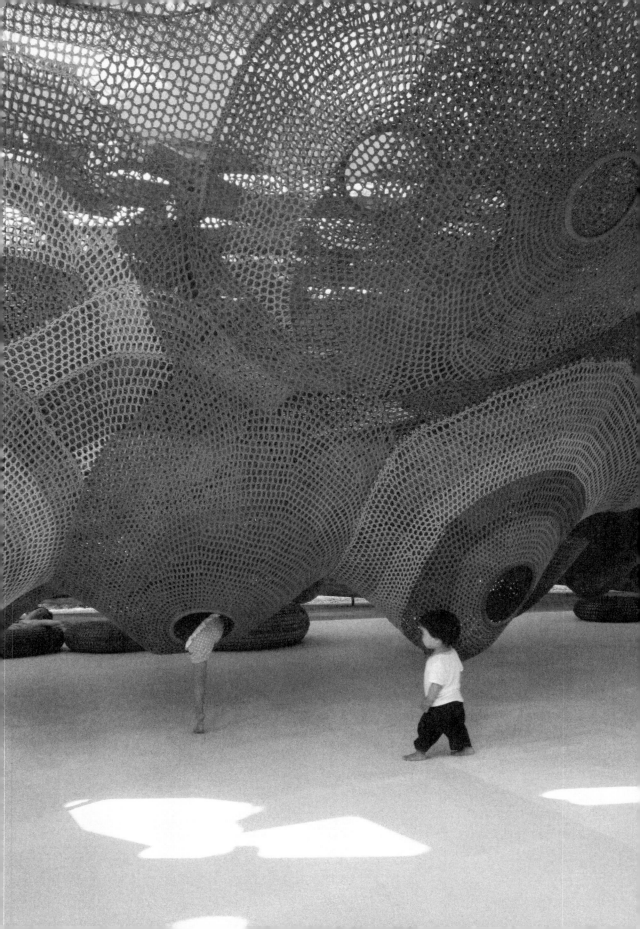

Acknowledgments

This book is a companion volume, in that it follows and expands my initial *American Playgrounds: Revitalizing Community Space* (2005). It is a pleasure to work again with my earlier publisher, University Press of New England. Their team, including editor-in-chief Phyllis Deutsch and director Michael Burton, has been diligent and supportive. I am fortunate to have such dedicated people overseeing this project. It is gratifying that Ellen Wicklum, formerly at UPNE and the person who acquired the first book, remains a cheerleader from afar.

Chip McGee, Grace Ong-Yan, Bob Solomon, and Audra Wolfe read all or parts of the manuscript. I am deeply thankful for their extensive help in shaping the final outcome. I regret and am saddened that Marvin Bressler, who read my previous book manuscripts, is no longer alive to offer his witty and profound comments.

Ellen B. H. Sandseter (Trondheim), Elger Blitz (Amsterdam), Naomi Pollock (Tokyo), Isami Kinoshita (Tokyo), Javier Malo de Molina (Madrid), and Helle Nebelong (Copenhagen) were especially kind in escorting me through their respective cities. I owe them all many thanks for helping me gain insights I could never have gotten in other ways.

I have badgered many people for information. No one disappointed me, and often they offered sager thoughts than I even knew to request. I humbly thank the following scientists, designers, art historians, librarians, play advocates, astute observers: Gamze Abramov, Yossi Abramov, Vito Acconci, Michel van Ackere, Monica Adams, Karen Adolph, Tim Ahern, Lisa Albin, Joan Almon, Robert Aspinall, Sarah Weidner Astheimer, Randi Augenstein, Russell Baldon, Connie Ban, Adrian Benepe, Amy Berlin, Jay Beckwith, Chris Berthelsen, Pål Bøyesen, Geir Brendeland, David Brownlee, Donne Buck, Jane Clark Chermayeff, Mark Christensen, Deborah Cordonnier, Amy Crews, Scott Dahlman, Sharon Gamson Danks, Richard Dattner, Adele Diamond, Judy Diamond, Patty Donald, Tim Ebikon, Iben Falconer, Alexander Filip and the staff of the CPSC, Karyn Flynn, M. Paul Friedberg, Svane Frode, Julie Gawendo, Lisa Gelfand, Cynthia Gentry, Tim Gill, Alex Gilliam, Phil Ginsburg, Jean Grossman, Denis Guzzo, Yashar Hanstad, Roger Hart,

Marit Haugen, Teri Hendy, Joy Hendry, Peter Heuken, Mark Horton, Walter Hood, Pei Hsiang, Jennifer Isacoff, Masako Irie, Paige Johnson, Anna Kassman-McKerrell, Sekiichi Kato, Barbara Kaucky, Linda Keane, Rose Kelly, H. Nyunny Kim, Jeff Kingston, Eriko Kinoshita, Steven Koch, Carol Krinsky, Reinhard Kropf, James Lambiasi, Martin Van Der Linden, Charles MacAdam, Toshiko MacAdam, Shuto Machko, Nancy Gonzalez Madynski, John Medina, Shilpa Mehta. Jayne Merkel, Mary Miss, Jørgen Moe, Maki Onishi, Michiko Ono Paddock, Matt Passmore and Rebar Group, Césare Peeren, Jane Perry, Linda Pollak, Nancy Pressman, Todd Rader, Chris Reed, Brent Richter, Jackie Safier, Katherin Sauerwein, Martha Schwartz, Sherry Schweighardt, Martin Seligman, Ken Smith, Bernard Spiegal, Siv Helene Stangeland, Lisa Switkin, Sarah Tabata, Riho Tanaka, Takaharu Tezuka, Yui Tezuka, Karl-Chirstian Thies, Meredith Thomas, Martha Thorne, Nancy Thorne, Matt Urbanski, David Walker, Peter Walker, Sam Wang, Nicky Washida, Bill Whitaker, Robert Whitaker, Clément Willemin, Penny Wilson, Katie Winter, Rob Wilson, Carla Yanni, and Dan Zohar.

Amy Ogata, Nicholas Day, and Sam Abrams have each written works that set a context to make my job easier. Firestone Library at Princeton University has been my perfect haven in which to write.

My family continues to nurture me. I know that I can always—and do constantly—rely on Jon Solomon's critical perceptions, shrewd sense of design, and capacity to bring people together for my benefit; Debra Solomon's encouragement and insistence that I write a second playground book; Nicole Scheller's insightful viewpoints from the vantage of a good teacher; and Gil Carmel's smart assessments of computer games and play.

Grandchildren Maggie, Noa, and Adam show me the wonder that comes from well-crafted play sites. It is a thrill to spend time with them (on and off playgrounds) and satisfying to see how their parents are enabling them to have joyful childhoods.

I happily dedicate this book to my husband, Bob Solomon. He has cooked a lot of linguini with green beans when I have been away and taken superb photos when we have traveled together. I am lucky to have such an understanding, generous, and talented spouse.

The Science of Play

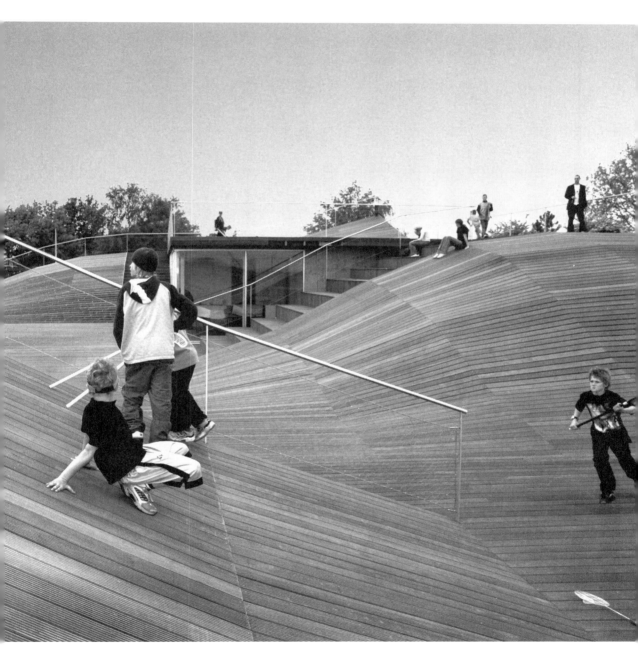

Introduction

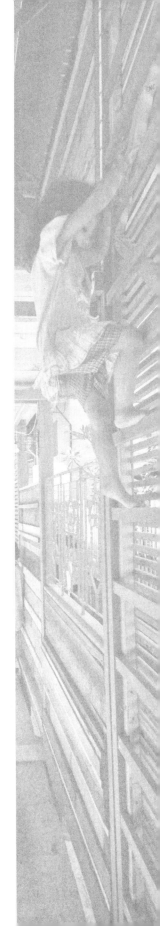

ORGET PLAY. Dismiss, for a moment, any belief that play is valuable for children. Ignore any of the places where it could occur. Put old notions aside so that we can take a fresh look at the American playground and use bold innovative strategies to improve it.

We need to think audaciously because current discussion about play, play value, and play spaces has reached an impasse. The definition of play remains fluid. It could be teachers guiding an open-ended and unstructured exercise. Or it could be pursuits that are engaging and that elicit pleasurable emotions.[1] It could be activities without goals, whimsical ways to participate in new actions.[2] Behavioral scientists support a definition that describes internal motivation without a specific purpose; the means have greater value than the end product.[3] Play workers in the United Kingdom may have the most sustainable outlook, one that blends well with the reality of outdoor space. They maintain that play is action that is "freely chosen, personally directed and intrinsically motivated."[4]

In contemporary American culture, play is "either ignored or idealized."[5] Assessments of play value sit on a broad spectrum: one play proponent "holds that depriving children and youth of play turns them into mass murderers."[6] On the opposite side are those who feel that play is expendable, especially from school-day activities. Play advocates may be overzealous in "attributing benefits [to] play," while play deriders may be too swift to discount the usefulness of play.[7] On both sides of the debate, anecdotes often take the place of evidence.

Even pronouncements from academic circles yield conflicting results. Play is contrasted with directives or school testing. The book *Play = Learning*, which published papers from an earlier conference of the same name, imparts comprehensive documentation of play theories and studies but leans toward guided play as the preferred prototype. We all want to believe that play bolsters language development, aids conflict resolution, and enhances the ability to understand others, but some researchers argue that "any hard evidence for how play in itself contributes to many of these developments is not easy to provide."[8] One diligent investigator says that "the empirical record supporting the unequivocal value of play is weak."[9] Play's role in supporting problem solving and creativity, proposed in the 1970s, was not reproducible in double-blind experiments in the 1980s.[10] Free play can be useful if it means that children can be independent and if it allows for "social learning and physical exercise . . . [but the] educational (cognitive) benefits of free play with objects are probably exaggerated."[11] Play England, the remarkable advocacy and research association, issued a review of the literature that found a better link between play and motivation, emotion, and resilience than cognitive gain.[12]

The concept of play, with so many inconsistencies, can no longer be the sole justification for monetary expenditures on public spaces for children. Studying it exclusively is not rigorous enough to protect and enhance play spaces. Even Johan Huizinga's magisterial *Homo Ludens: A Study of the Play-Element in Culture* (1938, translated and published in English in 1949) is more philosophical than specific for our needs. We must shift the discussion so that people who commission playgrounds—and those who design them—will have suitable information with which to inform their decisions, and to extricate themselves from excessive worries about insurance costs or liability. To that end, this book makes an argument for American public play spaces, based on broad, systemic questions rather than nostalgia or wistful aspirations. What do kids need to thrive? What factors affect how children mature emotionally, socially, culturally? What type of experiences will help them become competent adults? How do we provide unpredictable daily occurrences that will enable kids to think through unexpected challenges? How can we prepare them to engage with a future we cannot envision?

Data drawn from the behavioral sciences (and, to a lesser degree, from the neurosciences) provide some useful starting points.[13] Recent studies, some of which are just in their infant stage, hint at the experiences kids need so that they can mature. Underlying these investigations is the concept that "the brain is more plastic and changeable, even in adulthood, than ever thought before."[14] We know that nature and nurture are interconnected; these links, once limited to theory, now can be measured with precise tools or mapped with sophisticated imaging. There is an interactive flux, flowing in both directions, between biology and experience.[15] These findings indicate that children should have as many varied and broad opportunities as possible.

This book, taking advantage of established and emerging information, integrates science and design so that any person—but particularly American urban policy-makers, designers, educators, and parents—will have a working knowledge of what kids might require to enhance their lives. The book provides a resource that illustrates what recent findings could look like when translated into real physical spaces. The goal is to apply new criteria to designs for children's outdoor space and to let a broad audience see that exciting results are attainable, attractive, and affordable.

This book demonstrates how architects and landscape architects, particularly in Europe and Japan, have embraced and, in some cases, already incorporated scientific hypotheses into their designs. Some of these designers are aware of current scientific thinking; others have relied on their own backgrounds and histories to create progressive designs that mesh well with scientific thought. These solutions reflect notions of national identity and conceptions of childhood that encourage innovative solutions for children. They show how an overarching allegiance to a common good sustains a creative approach to play, one that promotes artists joining the design process.

While Americans tend to devise ways to protect children, we should be aware of options in other parts of the world and look to those models, which invest trust in young people, for approaches to children's outdoor activities. Foreign solutions for public space often avoid the rigidity and predictability of traditional playground equipment. Their constructions are cost effective, usually sustainable and accessible, and frequently unique. By bringing attention to these success stories, this book hopes to fill voids that designers and patrons know exist. Architects and landscape architects need a framework to go to for advice on playgrounds. Patrons need a resource that encourages them to initiate innovative projects. This book hopes to satisfy both requirements, wherever possible using examples of universal design that are accessible and welcoming.

Time is of the essence. Large American cities, which frequently allocate $2 to $3 million to upgrade a playground, are currently getting very little return on their investment. The same is true in midsize cities and towns, where $400,000 to $750,000 has become the norm. Compared with the cost of erecting a school or library, the playground could be a bargain if these same sites were tools for stimulating children's daily lives and forging stronger intergenerational communities. Unlike the school or library, most playground equipment is expected to last only fifteen years. This is a shockingly short life span. Our hope should be to find solutions that can be easily renewed or possibly last longer.[16]

American children inhabit a world that has shrunk to home, school, and planned activities. A proliferation of indoor pay-to-play businesses beckon. A focus on indoor activities has been visible for at least a decade. In 2004,

Wisk laundry detergent helped to underwrite a careful survey of mothers' and children's outdoor play which found that 70 percent of the responding moms had played outdoors every day as children, whereas only 31 percent of their own children did.[17] The soap maker, which allied its report with its own America Needs Dirt campaign, feared that kids were not playing outside and no longer getting dirty.

We offer children and their families few inducements to include public space in their rounds, and they become increasingly "absent from the community."[18] The physical state of American play areas deters visitors and aids the antiplay voices. Designs, endlessly replicated across America, suggest that kids are not doing anything constructive. To a certain extent, that is true. Spiffy recent installations contribute little to children's maturity or their sense of independence. One or two pieces of bland metal or plastic equipment dominate the sites. These objects are often single-directional — forcing kids to go up, across, and down. A few additional supplements, such as low faux rocks or a restyled jungle gym that is close to the ground, do little to vary scenarios or offset the static ensemble. All the time we hear that children are living overly structured lives, yet we typically offer them close-ended play that reinforces the burden.[19]

The terrain of patronage is enlarging, thereby creating a shift that could alter the status quo. Parks departments in San Francisco and Chicago are expanding their mission to include adult exercise sections or dog runs adjacent to playgrounds. Both options enliven outdoor venues. New York is among a number of densely populated cities that are beginning to reopen schoolyards to the public during nonschool hours, saving valuable resources, providing more neighborhood-friendly locations for play, and setting a tone for valuing community street life.[20] Municipal transportation agencies are commissioning public spaces that include activities for children. The roof for the San Francisco TransBay Transit Center (Cesar Pelli, architect and PWP Landscape Architecture), a hub for trains, streetcars, and buses that will open in 2017, will cater to leisure and its plans include a dedicated play zone. This ecologically diverse five-acre park, sixty feet above ground, will be the center of a burgeoning residential and commercial scheme.

Play spaces can carry marketing cachet and economic potential. Midcentury shopping malls used to embed a few play pieces into a central interior space; even earlier, in the 1920s, department stores provided supervised play spaces.[21] Recently some retail developers have taken advantage of adjacent exterior space to establish public play spaces that are attractive to a variety of ages and enhance the streetscape. Adults participate because these

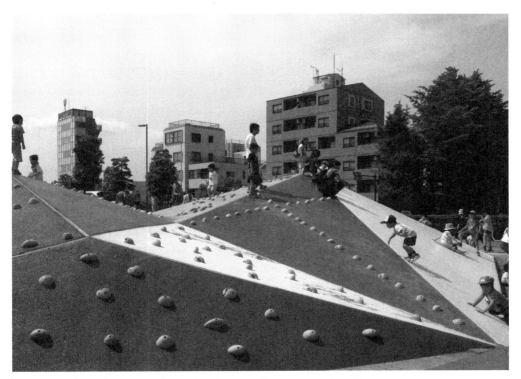

FIGURE I.1 | *Earthscape Landscape Architecture, play space on edge of Lazona Kawasaki Plaza shopping mall (Ricardo Bofill Taller de Arquitectura), Tokyo, 2006. Author's photograph, 2013.*

are disarming activities, not because parents feel that they must vigilantly watch their offspring. Toshiko Horiuchi MacAdam created a net structure (2012) for the retail district of Zaragoza, Spain. In Tokyo, local landscape firm Earthscape designed a multiage piece for the enormous Lazona Kawasaki Plaza (Ricardo Bofill Taller de Arquitectura) shopping mall. Located on a street corner and next to both a surface parking lot for the shopping center and its enclosed garage, the playground is a series of hard rubber folded planes. People of all ages run up to the top of one pyramid, then swoop down into another before starting another ascent; one surface is flat to allow sliding into sand at the bottom.

Residential developers, who represent an industry that at times has resisted integrating child-friendly spaces into their projects, are now looking to playgrounds as a marketing tool. In San Francisco, a developer hired PWP Landscape Architecture to envision a public park adjacent to a proposed residential project. PWP drew a four-thousand-square-foot "play garden" with sculpted rocks, sand, and running water where children might climb, splash, or socialize. Similarly, the developers of Northshore Hamilton Park, a mixed-use development on the site of the old Brisbane (Australia) wharfs, commissioned artist Fiona Foley (through Urban Art Projects) to design a playscape. Their goal was to enrich community gatherings and to boost sales. In Gloucestershire (UK), purchasers of upscale houses made a ruckus when a promised playground irritated the aesthetic taste of neighbors and the developer closed it off until the company could repaint it. When the delay did not quickly end, some resident parents let it be known that the playground was one of the reasons they had purchased homes in this subdivision.[22]

The healthcare industry is also taking notice. American pediatricians are finding themselves in a dual role as both advocates for and patrons of play spaces. Their professional association has issued major reports that urge parents to allow their children to have more unstructured free time. These reports recommend that pediatricians learn about the play resources in their communities so they can make recommendations to parents.[23] These are professionals who are familiar with the science of play; they grasp the significance of kids having opportunities for joyful nonacademic experiences. They are committed to increasing public play spaces, but they often have no idea of the implications for the built environment. They need to have more visual references, and they need to see what it would look like to apply their conclusions to groundbreaking designs.

In The Hague, in the Netherlands, a residential care facility (a type of assisted living mostly for elderly people) was built next to a public park (Billie Holiday Park, named for the adjacent street) that wasn't attracting many users. Once the building complex was completed, the municipal authorities recognized that an upgraded playground for families would be suitable and useful. Design firm Carve (founded by Elger Blitz and Mark van der Eng) came up with a single, multigenerational structure that is the new heart of the neighborhood.[24] The designers smartly provided a constructed "playhill" with seating ledges, bicycle racks, swings, sand, climbing frame, embedded trampolines, and a six-foot-high climbing wall. These nestle into a continuous surface; users have many options, and the overall amorphous shape fits snugly onto the land. Carve has shown how it is possible to create a striking object that appeals to children, offers them varied opportunities, and draws together a diverse population, all for a modest sum (less than half of what a small American city would pay for standard equipment and surfacing).[25] The park, once desolate, is now flourishing because so many people gravitate to this play piece.[26]

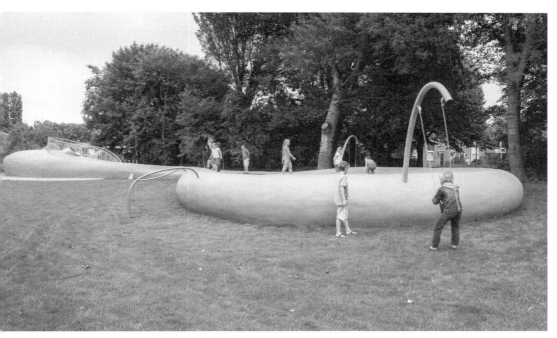

FIGURE I.2 | *Carve. Billie Holiday Park, The Hague, Netherlands, 2013. The materials for the play piece are reinforced concrete placed over geo-textile (for shape) and a metal frame. Courtesy of Carve.nl. Photograph by Marleen Beek, 2013.*

Caveats and Confidence

This book comes with a few caveats and a lot of optimism. This is a book that is largely about outdoor urban spaces (the World Bank estimates that more than 80 percent of Americans live in urban areas), primarily but not exclusively for children, and how those spaces might be improved. There is observational evidence that kids play longer and more complexly when they are outside.[27] This book does not, for the most part, address sports, games (unless they are spontaneous), or organized recreation. Wherever possible, it searches for multigenerational solutions and for ones that tap into the skills of artists of all stripes, including architects and landscape architects.

Since there is concern that biologists and neuroscientists have been too quick to make a connection between mammalian and human behavior, this book does not rely on animal studies for evidence.[28] Nor does this book contain an exhaustive discussion about achieving healthy bodies, combating obesity, or handling bullying; those concerns raise other issues that demand separate books with nuanced investigations.[29] Similarly, and because this is a book about public venues, it does not dwell on conversations about

how parents can love or be tender with their offspring. Other books investigate those issues.

Each chapter of this book highlights a different value that is missing in
most playgrounds: risk, mastery (with the possibility to fail on the way to
success), executive function (planning, problem solving, juggling working
memory), friendship (including having pals of differing ages), possible
exposure to nature, and rough-and-tumble play. These categories are not
arbitrary or definitive; they represent some of the topics that are most prevalent in contemporary discussions of child development, ones that also are
most adaptable to design programs. The choice of playground examples
was more subjective. Most of the playgrounds shown here exhibit multiple
characteristics; they represent a particular success but could easily fit into
several of the categories. To highlight the most approachable play spaces,
this book cites cases that have no admission cost; in a few instances, there is
an entry charge, but the design could be a prototype for another free, local
setting.

This is a positive moment for play spaces in America. There is a small
but growing backlash, evident since 2000, against the current state of affairs: patrons, administrators, and parents are ready to listen to novel ideas.
Having feared liability and insurance costs for too long, and realizing that
playgrounds are fast becoming an overpriced resource that adds little to a
community, some adults are willing to consider alternatives. Sales of Conn
and Hal Iggulden's *The Dangerous Book for Boys* and Gever Tulley's and Julie
Spiegler's *50 Dangerous Things (You Should Let Your Children Do)* evidence a
deep yearning for less constriction in children's lives.[30] Richard Louv's *Last
Child in the Woods* similarly hit a nerve. The greening schoolyards movement is gaining momentum.

We might be ready to hear a message that is relevant, even if it is almost
thirty years old. In 1985, architect Aase Eriksen, who practiced in both Denmark and the United States, wrote a prescient book entitled *Playground Design: Outdoor Environments for Learning and Development*. Eriksen bemoans
the state of American playgrounds. She observes that they are often empty,
too boring to hold the attention of children, and consequently derided as
frivolous by those who feel play is worthless. Her recommendations are
incisive: kids have a natural inclination to develop their own independence
and interests. We can encourage those by ditching age- segregated playgrounds and replacing them with "playscapes" (generalized play areas that
fit seamlessly into their surroundings) that can be community hubs as well
as environments that stimulate "the development of the child's physical,

emotional, social, and intellectual abilities."[31] She demands a varied experiential condition in which children can "explore and manipulate" the environment. She sees the nonschool use of schoolyards as essential for expanding the number of play sites.[32]

Eriksen knew, and we can learn, how outdoor spaces can aid in helping kids negotiate their way in the world. Using scientific information, we can reevaluate our current spaces and find ways to offer more variability and unexpected conclusions. Let's make sure that these reinvented spaces do their job well and in the most effective, exciting, responsible, and inexpensive way possible. Successful spaces cannot solve all of children's challenges, but they can provide chances for kids to mature, to grow emotionally, to become more competent and confident. We can no longer feign surprise that kids avoid playgrounds. We have curbed their excitement and fearlessness. We can, however, begin to reassess and redress the situation in hopes of providing more opportunities for kids and better spaces for us all.

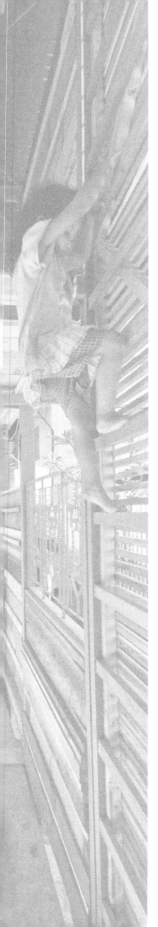

The Problem 4

WE LIVE IN UNCERTAIN TIMES, characterized by pressures to prepare our children for undefined future challenges. We are not the first generation to attempt to ready children for terrifyingly unknown events. In 1962, toy and playground manufacturer Creative Playthings published a catalog whose message could be speaking to our own plight. The catalog states that parents and teachers "are being called upon to prepare children for a world so radically new that we dare not forecast its direction, its technology, and its social organization."[1] The launch of Sputnik and the ongoing Cold War informed their unease; we have to confront even more startling technological breakthroughs, a more complex political landscape, and a physical environment that is more dense and urban.

The American playground today fails as a resource that could help kids mature or prepare for unidentified future ordeals. Unlike the exciting playgrounds of the 1950s and 1960s, best illustrated by Creative Playthings' Play Sculptures division, which commissioned artists to rethink the playground concept, today's typical American playground does a particularly bad job at preparing children for uncertainty. We find maintenance-free caged areas that emphasize safety more than critical thinking, smart reasoning, hopeful investigations, or thrilling adventures.

KFC + P

When we look at today's stock playground, we see an aesthetically unappealing place with few opportunities for personal exploration or social development. The equipment is predictable and demeaning. Almost any child can maneuver easily on it. There is no struggle or sense of accomplishment. Everyone succeeds, but the achievement does not have any triumph; it does not require any struggle or cooperation. No kid can really alter the environment. There is little chance that anyone will ever have a scraped knee or bruised elbow, minor injuries that used to indicate that a child had tried something new. A palette of lurid, jarring, and unnatural colors seem to scream to children that this is a jolly setting; the color choices seem to

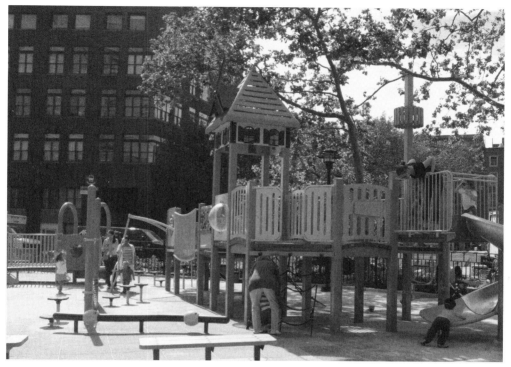

FIGURE 1.1 | *Pearl Street Playground, New York City, reconstructed and enlarged in 2012. A private grant of $2.1 million paid for this renovation. The fencing has become less intrusive than earlier play spaces, but the equipment remains banal and the surfacing is monotonous. The new plantings are outside the fence, close to the sidewalk, so they are out of reach for playground use. It is unclear why an adult is on this low equipment. Photograph by Robert S. Solomon, 2013.*

say that the play structure has already created the fun. Kids are not trusted to produce their own bliss.

The British have a nickname for this standard playground: "KFC," for kit, fence, and carpet.[2] American arrangements, which replicate the same dull ensemble, add another threat into the mix: parents. The banal end results of KFC + P mean that we deny children a chance to gain a small bit of independence, to learn a few skills, to meet peers and other generations, and even to get dirty.

Concerns about costs, including liability, drive many decisions about American playground design. Park departments and school boards purchase standard equipment, which they replace when it "looks old," because it meets their most pressing requirements: it has easy upkeep and it limits their liability. The plastic and metal products need little to no maintenance. To be doubly safe, some authorities shut them down after drizzle or fog because they fear that they may become slippery.

Manufacturers reassure clients that their products meet or exceed all federal guidelines, but the equipment is expensive because the liability cost is built into each sale; local patrons hope to effectively turn their legal concerns over to the manufacturers by buying off-the-shelf products. We have become an increasingly litigious people. Since the 1980s we have nurtured a culture of victimization.[3] Parents feel that the smallest injury can be blamed on someone other than their own child. The American legal system sometimes allows generous damages for an injury, and parents often pursue financial remuneration. In Europe or Japan there is minimal financial compensation; the legal system restricts tort damages. Instead, the European or Japanese child is expected to take stock of his actions and consider his own and communal safety.[4] After an accident, the European or Japanese child would probably say, "What did I do wrong?"; the American child (or his parents) might ask, "Where is my lawyer?"[5]

The difficulty with the American safety guidelines is that they address almost every possibility for injury, both minor and serious. The Consumer Product Safety Commission (CPSC) published its first "Handbook for Public Playground Safety" in 1981. Those federal "suggestions," as well as the more technical ones of the American Society for Testing and Materials (ASTM) that followed, continue to be updated and remain as effective as legislation. Insurance agents demand that their clients adhere to them. Even Teri Hendy, a highly respected playground consultant and an expert on safety who helped write the ASTM standards, says that these failed institutionally from the beginning because they tried to erase all risk.[6] She now believes that the ASTM should have focused only on preventing fatal, life-threatening, or debilitating injuries. She recognizes how attention to minor injuries has overwhelmed our requirements.[7] Other observers have noted that universally we tend to lump minor and major occurrences into a single category of "injuries."[8]

The CPSC guidelines demand regularity in the equipment that may itself be a type of hazard. Danish Landscape architect Helle Nebelong argues that the uniform spacing of the manufactured pieces, especially seen in stairs and horizontal ladders, lulls kids into expecting conformity and leaves them unprepared for having to deal with variation.[9] Children who have never had to assess their surrounds expect every rung of a ladder or a monkey bar to be uniformly separated. These kids have no capacity to make appropriate judgments when they face situations that have not been perfectly engineered. Neuroscientists Sandra Aamodt and Sam Wang add that American playground equipment fails to let children distinguish between what is safe and what is dangerous.[10]

Another paradox is that the federal American guidelines, which purport to cover everything, miss some real menaces. A glaring omission can be seen in the way the CPSC's "Public Playground Safety Handbook" (2008) addresses swings. They suggest a "use zone" of "6 feet in all directions from the perimeter of the equipment," with nothing within that six-foot radius. A change in surfacing color (for example, a large circle) will often identify the use zone. This solution makes sense on paper but means nothing to a toddler rushing through a playground to get from one activity to another. A more feasible solution would be to raise the swings onto a slightly higher plane (such as a low mound) to designate the use zone and to divert a small person, but that is not suggested or encouraged.

The federal guidelines do more than just ensure overbuilt, risk-avoidant equipment. By calling for age segregation, the guidelines reveal a disconnect between playground structure and current thinking on the pedagogy of play. Our playgrounds typically have one area for the two- to five-year-old set and a higher contraption for the five-to-twelve range. Manufacturers have recently added a category for babies, from six to twenty-three months, so we may begin to see a third area for the tinniest users. Although there is a certain logic in separating the smallest most vulnerable users from older participants, contemporary educators and psychologists look to interactions between age groups as the way that older kids push younger ones to mature. They cite the writings of Lev Vygotsky (1896–1934) as their source.[11] His teachings have been influential since the 1980s, in spite of the fact that he died decades ago and his works were unknown in the West until the 1960s.[12]

The age distinctions on today's playgrounds hark to the 1950s, when child psychologists Jean Piaget and Erik Erikson, both of whom emphasized the successive stages of child development, were the most audible voices.[13] Today there is growing unease with Piaget's theories because scientists have shown that not all children go through these predetermined stages.[14] We now believe that older kids can pull along younger ones ("zone of proximal development" is the Vygotsky term) and help them to achieve a bit more socially and cognitively than they might on their own or solely with peers.

Fans of current playground design have always had a fallback position: the equipment may be dull, but at least it provides a way for kids to experience heavy-duty exercise. Recent research shows that that position, too, may be untenable. A limited preliminary study shows that the mere presence of equipment does not increase physical activity, possibly because children spend time waiting in line or because there isn't much opportunity to use it.[15] Today's equipment is good for handgrip and hand coordination; it does not address upper body, core strength, or conditioning.[16] Children need exercises that activate locomotive skills, such as running, jumping, hopping, and skipping. Government guidelines published by the Centers for Disease Control and Prevention implore parents to see that kids get aerobic exercise in addition to bone strengthening and muscle strengthening activities.[17]

We need innovative solutions, yet playground patrons often forgo architects, landscape architects, or other artists, because they believe (mistakenly) that their expertise and their designs will be too expensive. Eliminating design professionals contributes to bland results. The good news is that, when they are brought in, designers—who are also cognizant of potential lawsuits—are enhancing projects without elevating costs. It is a "win-win" situation for all involved, with the results suggesting that we might see more creative designs that do more and cost less than the ordinary stock items. Jackie Safier, the donor for the Helen Diller Playground (2011) at Dolores Park in San Francisco, where landscape architect Steve Koch altered the positioning of off-the-shelf equipment and mixed it with pieces of his own design, wisely states, "Spend money on the designer and it will pay off in the end."[18]

Fencing

While the familiarity of standard-issue playground equipment may leave children feeling bored, the high fence that typically surrounds a play area makes it explicit that child's play is an activity restricted to firm boundaries. It circumscribes their actions, making sure that their play world is confined. The playground has come to resemble a caged island, one that reinforces the notion that children are being raised "in captivity."[19]

The ever-present fence might be understandable if its intent were to keep small children away from traffic. Cars pose a very real threat to youngsters, and we, of course, have to do everything possible to keep small fry from going into the street. But fences are hardly the only solution. Landscaping, often with thick shrubbery, achieves the same results without appearing to place kids in "jail." An alternative approach retains the fence but masks it with plants or architectural elements. Architect Linda Pollak (Marpillero

Pollak Architects) is someone who points to untapped possibilities for in-corporating a resting place with benches or adapting a climbing or swinging apparatus into an enclosure.[20]

Today, with playgrounds often quite far from streets, the high fences mirror parental fears more of trespassers coming in than of kids getting out. A New York City municipal ordinance makes it an offense to enter a play-ground without a child in tow. Other cities have similar ordinances or have warnings to the same effect. Signs on gates reinforce the message; they not too subtly remind parents to be diligent, to be suspicious of a single adult.

It is good news for society and parents that worrying about playground abductions is a gratuitous gesture. It turns out that "stranger danger" is a very real paranoia, but that the underlying fears that provoke it are not realistic. Historian Steven Mintz, an authority on the history of American childhood, points out that these fears emerged first in the 1970s and do not seem to be abating.[21] He uses the sociological term "moral panic" to explain how overwrought fears replace legitimate concerns, eventually immersing us in a culture of fear. According to Mintz, absurd but prevalent conclusions about safety and risk take hold and force the hand of politicians; fear rather than facts dominates how policy is written.[22]

The possibility that a stranger will abduct a child from a playground is infinitesimally small. Abductors are usually people children know, not strangers.[23] The last nationwide statistic for abductions dates from 1999;[24] that year, there were 262,215 abductions. (Follow up research started only in 2010 and has not concluded.) Of those, strangers or slight acquaintances were the perpetrators in only 115 events.[25] One writer puts that number in context as follows: for the 59 million American children who were age four-teen or younger in 1999, the risk that any one of them would be abducted by a stranger was 1 in 655,555. The same author notes that, less than five years later (2003), 285 children (younger than fourteen) drowned in swimming pools, and 2,408 died in automobile crashes. Doing the math, he concludes that a child is much "more likely to die in a car crash than [to] be abducted by a stranger."[26] Even though car fatalities have mercifully fallen (1140 in 2011, the most recent year studied), the statistics still validate the view of another observer, who notes that we respond to certain names—Etan Patz, Polly Klaas, Madeleine McCann—because abductions and killings by strangers are such a rarity. If they weren't so unusual, we would have too many names to remember.[27] In each of those horrible instances, the children were walk-ing on a street or sleeping in bed, not snatched from a playground.

An irony is that parents are risking traffic accidents as they drive kids around because they are not comfortable leaving them alone at a play-ground.[28] It may be that playgrounds are like airplanes in the 1950s and 1960s: countless adults feared flying despite the fact that getting to the air-port in a car was statistically a greater risk. Today, parents fear playgrounds even though the risk of taking a child there by automobile is more danger-ous than being at the play spot.

We are, furthermore, instilling unfounded fears in many kids. Pediatri-cian and public health physician Robert Whitaker has observed that kids pick up on the fear of their parents and wonder why they should go to a place that makes the adults so anxious.[29] Children have caught on to their parents' unease and have developed their own troubled views. In a survey in the United Kingdom, almost half the parents of seven- to fourteen-year-olds said that it is unsafe for them to let their children outside without adult supervision. Half of them (one-quarter of those polled) believed the immediate threat to be abduction. They have conveyed this fear to their kids: 48 percent of seven- to ten-year-olds agree that they need an adult nearby when they play outside. This number decreases only to 30 percent as they reach ages ten to fourteen.[30] More brazen children in Japan, who see the absurdity of overprotection and constant monitoring, will mock these by playing a game they call "stranger danger" or will play in a way that will intentionally take them out of the view of the mounted surveillance cameras.[31]

Kenneth R. Ginsburg, the lead author of an American Academy of Pedi-atrics report on play, sees more pragmatic reasons to stop overemphasizing the danger of abduction to children. He astutely reasons that kids may have real emergencies—sickness, an accident, being lost—that require them to reach out to strangers for assistance. Not doing so might further endanger them. Parents who demand that their offspring never talk to a stranger may be denying their children a way to seek real help when they need it.[32] Per-haps we have to give children different kinds of information, so that they can determine who might be dangerous or who might be a benign, even helpful, presence. That training could start at a more open playground.

By blocking single, older, or childless adults from playgrounds, we are limiting the possibility (and further justification for large monetary expen-ditures) that playgrounds could be community hubs. We are destroying the chance that a playground could be a "third space" or "third place," sites where people return over and over again to hang out, find fellowship, and gain a sense of community.[33] Community means more than coming together several times a year. It means knowing your neighbors, seeing them often.

The findings of sociologist Eric Klinenberg show that the formation of social capital is more than a nicety or a sweet notion of camaraderie. At times of natural disaster, the sense of shared spaces and of folks watching out for and helping each other can have an impact on survival. Klinenberg examined the role of informal associations in determining who died in a July heat wave that swept Chicago in 1995. In a comparison of two poor, crime-ridden sections of the city, Klinenberg found that the elderly were much more likely to survive in the neighborhood with a strong social infra-structure.[34] We have to consider how open playgrounds could contribute to fostering that type of human foundation.

Carpet

A third feature of almost all American playgrounds is a flat, poured-in-place, rubber ground covering known as a "unitary covering," or, more col-loquially in Britain, a "carpet." This ubiquitous surface reinforces the sense that playgrounds are risk-free, and, above all, clean. It is also expensive and can double the cost of a playground without contributing to what children can do. Kids cannot move it, mold it, or reconfigure it.

Playground carpets were originally introduced for children's protection. And indeed, modern surfacing is significantly safer than the asphalt or con-crete that once were the surface material for playgrounds. Head injuries, the greatest threat to kids, have almost vanished since the late 1970s. That is no inconsequential feat. The question now is how to maintain the current level of protection while simultaneously introducing variety and lowering the cost.[35]

Safety surfacing is, by now, taken for granted—so much so that there is a possibility that rubber surfacing, not unlike fencing, is a component that is chosen "as much on the basis of belief as on analysis."[36] Most falls and injuries today have an impact on upper limbs. David Ball, at the Centre for Decision Analysis and Risk Management at Middlesex University (UK), feels that the surfacing has not done anything to prevent injuries to these upper extremities.[37] The CPSC, which admits that no surfacing will prevent all injuries, accepts several loose-fill options, including wood chips or wood mulch, pea gravel, sand, or shredded tires. All of these create varied surfaces and offer shock absorption. They do require maintenance and refilling.[38]

Sand, if selected carefully, holds the greatest possibility for an inexpen-sive surface kids can play on that addresses both severe head injuries and some limb fractures. David Spease, a landscape architect and playground safety specialist, has done testing that shows that sand may be a more effective cushioning substance than originally thought. After seeing that the CPSC's guidelines reduced the permissible heights for falls on sand from five feet to four, Spease tested a particular mixture — lapis sand — for safety. It "contains limestone and sea shells and is frequently used for aquariums. It has rounded edges rather than sharp corners that you typically find in crushed stone products, and most of the particle sizes are about the same. It is kind of like really, really small pea stone." Spease found that it could cushion a fall from a ten-foot drop, allowing for the possibility of higher places to play and more varied surfaces on which to land.[39] A ten-foot drop onto sand would also ally American playgrounds with the reality of German playgrounds, which have adhered to that standard without severe consequences.[40]

The absence of sand and dirt compounds the sterility of the American playground. Many American cities are choosing to forgo sand or water, because they are considered "health risks" — which presumably means the possible appearance of stray hypodermic needles or cat feces. Here, too, fear may be dictating policy. It may come as a surprise that a study from Australia (a culture not too different from our own) shows that the occurrence of hidden needles or syringes in public sandboxes is extremely low;[41] the threat of these amounts almost to an "urban legend." The cat issue may not be as rare, but there are simple solutions that prevent sand from being a health risk. The Japanese are not alarmed by animal excrement; the last person to leave a public park simply puts the cover on the sandbox.[42] There should be equally uncomplicated ways to protect larger expanses of sand surfaces.

The sand- and dirt-free playground has become so ubiquitous that many children now shudder at the thought of getting filthy or having fun in the mud. In 2012 a mud and obstacle race for adults in the Bronx, New York, included a segment at the end for kids. The organizers invited children into the mud pit. Some refused to participate; an announcer told them not to "be afraid to get dirty." The kids prevailed, and the few who did finally participate ventured in "as fastidiously as wading egrets."[43] It is likely that they had been trained by parents who expect to find their children clean when picking them up from preschool or the park. In Norway, by contrast, adults often worry if their children are too spotless at the end of the day. In Japan there are at least five preschools that use mud play as the centerpiece of the daily curriculum.[44]

The American aversion to dirt may have larger consequences, which go beyond the realm of recreation. Mary Ruebush, who has a Ph.D. in immunoparasitology and who once found one of her children munching on horse manure after he crawled out of her view, has directly faced the importance of dirt in her book *Why Dirt Is Good*. She cogently argues that small children put things into their mouths because their bodies need a way to boost their immune systems, something that occurs with repeated exposure to "dirt." She defines dirt as anything or any place — not just soil — filled with germs. If kids get to taste dirt at an early age, it triggers immune responses. The young body "gets better, faster, and more specific" in attacking germs.[45] According to Ruebush, kids' bodies need constant exposure and retraining in order to stay healthy.[46]

Drs. Joel V. Weinstock (Tufts Medical Center) and David Elliott (University of Iowa) present equally compelling information about the usefulness of wormlike creatures called helminths, "intestinal worms [that] have been all but eliminated in developed countries." These worms rarely cause disease; indeed, they can trigger positive immune responses.[47] Weinstock argues that "children should be allowed to go barefoot in the dirt, play in the dirt, and not have to wash their hands when they come in to eat."[48] Weinstock and Ruebush provide arguments that make ridiculous a Minnesota state senator who introduced a bill to mandate daily cleaning of "all surfaces children touch" in playgrounds.[49]

Parents

Parents used to be on the sidelines of playgrounds. Now they are front and center, often hovering over young (or not-so-young) children. They are there to watch every move and frequently can be seen tailing their children on the equipment. The class differences in parenting that Annette Lareau recorded in her book *Unequal Childhoods* do not appear in parents' behavior on playgrounds. Shrinking family size, with fewer older siblings to help parents keep an eye on small fry, exacerbates the situation.[50] The phenomenon of parents inserting themselves into activities they never previously entered is becoming universal. In Norway and the Netherlands, a small number of parents are clinging to their kids; Japan has even coined their own term: "Monster Parents." These changes are strikingly new in those countries, and still relatively rare.[51]

Hovering is especially apparent in the United States and the United Kingdom. An extreme example occurred on an English playground, a facility that is fully staffed and that organizes sessions only for children. The mayor has stated that "several parents had invited themselves in and were then making a nuisance of themselves, interfering with what staff were doing" and (outrageously) "disciplining other people's children."[52] At that point, the play workers demanded the parents leave. The parents had apparently not respected the rules and boundaries of the playground and felt that they should have a say in their children's, and their neighbors' childrens', activities.

Some parents may feel they have to elevate play into drills that are akin to what they expect from school. They orchestrate their children's fun into a series of commands so that play time is not "wasted time." Parents who push academic achievement at an early age, and enroll three-year-olds in "drill and kill" academic preparation, are usually not aware of the possibility that their children might later have impaired motivation or poor discipline.[53]

There are other reasons that parents hover or are overly involved in how children play. One educator believes that attachment parenting, advocated by William and Martha Sears and based on earlier work by John Bowlby, has gone awry.[54] Sociologist Barry Glassner, historian Steven Mintz, and Judith Warner (author of *Perfect Madness: Motherhood in the Age of Anxiety*) speak with a common voice in explaining contemporary parenthood. Each sees a society in which parents feel so unable to control the events around them that they focus on perfecting and controlling their children. They overmanage their children because that is the one remaining arena where they can exercise real authority.[55] During economic downturns that make backsliding ever more difficult to avoid, parents micromanage their children to ensure (they believe) their future success. All three authors agree on the 1970s as the time of a shift in parental attitudes toward risk and safety, perhaps because of a stagnant economy.[56]

It may not be coincidental that parental hovering and fear of strangers surfaced at about the same time. The inauguration of the National Electronic Injury Surveillance System in 1970 (redesigned in 1978) most likely elevated parental angst. Throughout its history, epidemiologists have maintained that this data (based on a "probability sample" from one hundred hospitals with twenty-four-hour emergency room services) has been able to distinguish between minor and serious events,[57] but that has not been communicated well to the public. Parents believe that the accidents are becoming more prevalent and more severe. As a result, fears of death by injury or abduction become very real to adults who do not receive counterbalancing information. Wendy Grolnick, a childhood development specialist at Clark University who has extensively studied parenting, has a keen appraisal. She feels that parents try naturally and instinctively to protect their young. Her most recent work shows that parents become more intrusive and protective when they perceive a threat to their child.[58]

Injuries

Parents become justifiably upset when they read undifferentiated data that tells that there are 200,000 injuries on American public playgrounds per year. Those numbers do not distinguish between injuries such as a broken arm and a cracked skull, whereas the CPSC report on playground hazards has an age range of fourteen months to twenty-one years. We might wonder why the age limit is so high, when most children age out of playgrounds before they become teens; even the equipment specifies an upper age of twelve. We should also put the 200,000 injuries into a meaningful context: only four percent are hospitalized. To gain perspective, we need to know that 100,000 children under five require emergency room visits each year after falling down steps.[59] We can see that the percentage of injuries is much higher on stairs than playgrounds because the population for stairs (only those under five years old) is a discrete sample, whereas the playground data is much less exclusive.

Fatalities in public playgrounds in the United States and Europe are noticeably (and thankfully) very low.[60] In Europe the number is so small that it is not possible to generalize among causes; one researcher thinks that most of these tragic outcomes result from home equipment.[61] In the United States, twelve thousand children (age zero to nineteen) die of all types of injuries each year.[62] The most recent CPSC data covers deaths on playground equipment between 2001 and 2009. Over that eight-year period, forty deaths occurred.[63] The median age was four years. We should never minimize the tragedy of any death on the playground, but we need to take a close look at these sad occurrences. Twenty-seven of them were hangings or asphyxiations (none of which were deemed intentional). Most were caused by "secondary products," such as ropes, dog leashes, or jump ropes; two were related to clothing, possibly indicating that draw-strings — now forbidden by a CPSC ruling (16 CFR 1120) of 2011 that prohibits them on upper-body outerwear — could be in circulation as hand-me-downs. The remaining thirteen were head or neck injuries from falls (seven); product breakage (one); tipovers of swings sets (two), falls (two, one of which did not show traumatic injury); and one crash of an all-terrain vehicle being driven by a twenty-one-year-old.

Counterintuitively, overprotection does not necessarily eliminate danger.[64] Minor to moderate injuries will occur whether parents are standing over their kids or drinking a coffee nearby. A Harvard Medical School study in 2000 looked at playground injuries and found that the presence of adults did not change the outcomes.[65] And, in fact, American parents have unwittingly upset the design elements that used to deter children from being in situations where they don't belong. Landscape architect Paul Friedberg notes that designing a rung or step high above the ground was once an efficient way to keep small children off equipment meant for older kids.[66] Today, however, we see how parents will often place a young child on the high rung, or go down a corkscrew slide with a little one on their lap. Children fall, or parents get stuck on a turn and children's legs or arms get broken.[67] In such cases, there is a good possibility that the child's family will lodge a complaint and/or initiate a lawsuit and that very quickly the equipment will be deemed "unsafe" and will be removed.

The words of British post–World War II playground reformer Lady Allen of Hurtwood seem apt: "It is better to risk a broken leg than a broken spirit. A leg can always mend. A spirit may not."[68] Without making light of injuries, parents should remember that broken arms are usually the worst injuries that can result on a playground. Where there are broken limbs, kids recover quickly; fractures frequently need to be set and do not need surgery. Such injuries are much more minor than similar ones in adults.[69] Perception of healthcare options in the United States might drive many parents away from Lady Allen's position. The conventional wisdom is that children below the Medicaid line have no access to free medical care; in fact, they (and frequently those two or three times over the level of the poverty threshold) can receive treatment through Medicaid or through Child Help Plus (CHP).[70] The Affordable Care Act may fill in the gap for middle-class families that have been underinsured. These issues do not arise in Europe, the United Kingdom, or Japan, where there is universal public healthcare.

How Did We Get to This Mess?

We spend a lot of time talking about creating "place"—a sense that settings are indigenous, and specific—and yet our playgrounds are generic. Keen observer Nicholas Day sums up the situation: "Today, walking on a children's playground is like exiting the interstate. Regardless of where you are, you see the exact same thing."[71] We have to consider if this is a new phenomenon, or whether it has just become more apparent. It may be a mixture of both, with a history of uniformity in the late nineteenth century, inspired and artist-driven designs at midcentury, and decline for the last thirty years.

Reformers, who sought to aid and orchestrate the lives of the waves of new immigrants who landed on American shores in the early twentieth century, were the first to push playgrounds into a public realm. A symbol of how our government could protect and nurture its youngest citizens, early Reform era playgrounds offered extensive programming. During the first decades of the twentieth century, playgrounds were supposed to shield children from the hazards of the street; offer them advanced physical fitness opportunities; promote acculturation for immigrants; or provide a distinct place where children could, according to John Dewey, do "their own work." Reform era playgrounds were ambitious, far exceeding our own definition of what constitutes a play space. They often had a field house with showers and bathrooms, a library and/or dental clinic, playing fields, and running track. What we would call the equipment was the "apparatus" of ladders and slides.[72] To our contemporary eyes, some of this metal climbing equipment looks both flimsy and dizzyingly high. This exercise equipment was available for adults as well as children.[73] There is some indication that children abandoned Reform era playgrounds, which had gender- and age-segregated spaces, in the teens of the twentieth century, into order to seek "danger and adventure."[74]

The child-centric public play space emerged when the Reform era began to ebb and when the immigrant population had become accustomed to American ways. Playground equipment, specifically for children, came into its own in the 1930s. These pieces were usually plain independent swings or slides or seesaws, most of which were metal. There were fantastical and themed pieces, too, but the underlying form was usually swing, slide, or occasional child-powered merry-go-round.

Inventive playgrounds—often designed by architects, landscape architects, or sculptors—exemplified the period after World War II. Staff and programs were still critical to keeping children entertained. The optimism, economic growth, increased leisure time, and the sheer number of children born of the baby boom altered American society and encouraged investment in public recreation. During this time, educators looked to "open-ended objects that might stimulate original thinking."[75] They saw that the young boomers who were becoming elementary school students needed opportunities to be creative. American artists, who pioneered and led the world by using abstraction as their language during the 1950s and 1960s, saw how their outlook meshed with America's perception that creativity in the Cold War was a democratic ideal.[76]

In 1953 the Museum of Modern Art (MoMA), *Parents Magazine* (started in 1926 by psychologists interested in child rearing),[77] and toy and play-ground manufacturer Creative Playthings sponsored a seminal playground competition. Winning entries, which Creative Playthings promised to put into production, showed that artists could create interesting, aesthetically worthwhile play equipment. In one of the winning designs, children played in an abstract playhouse with a sand floor and exposed rebar "monkey bars" for the roof; another winner had low ramps for running, jumping, or wiggling though small tunnels. The MoMA, *Parents Magazine*, and Creative Playthings venture may have been the largest and most advertised example of the midcentury impulse toward creative play; it has sometimes overshadowed the many other architects and sculptors who were soon producing unusual play settings. Their endeavors elevated the appreciation of the child's material world; children were entrusted to make educated choices about their own safety. Adults accepted that kids were able to negotiate challenges. Parents tolerated a certain amount of risk.

The MoMA exhibition brought an alliance of artists and playground design to the attention of the public. A playground, designed by architect Louis Kahn and sculptor Isamu Noguchi beginning in 1961, further cemented the collaborative notion for playgrounds.[78] Together, the two created a total environment for play in New York City that was different from anything seen previously. Art patron Audrey Hess, who had earlier chosen Noguchi for an unexecuted playground adjacent to the United Nations building, brought these two men together. She wanted this playground to be a memorial to her aunt, Adele R. Levy, a noted art patron. By commissioning an architect at a smaller scale and a sculptor at a larger scale than either usually encountered, Hess was ensuring an unusual design for the site in Riverside Park.

The two artists came up with a scheme that used mostly concrete; it descended over the three levels of the park but could not be seen by anyone driving along Riverside Drive. Multiple ramps organized the space. Filled with embankment slides, an amphitheater, truncated pyramids, and abstract concrete shapes, this playground plan became well known for the way its amenities meshed into the concrete surface; land forms became a permanent hardscape. It also became notorious for the negative reaction it ignited from neighbors who thought it would be too much of a draw for people from other neighborhoods. The playground, which was never executed (in large part because of neighborhood opposition), imprinted its environmental design on the minds of young designers.

In the late 1960s, architect Richard Dattner and landscape architect M. Paul Friedberg, working independently, rethought the Kahn-Noguchi

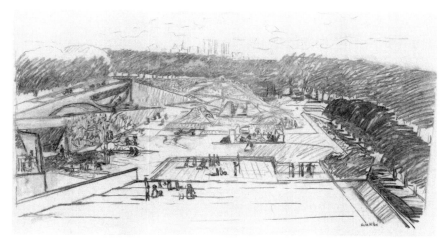

FIGURE 1.2 | *Louis I. Kahn, sketch for Adele R. Levy Playground (ca. 1966), New York. Kahn designed this unexecuted playground with sculptor Isamu Noguchi. Courtesy of the Louis I. Kahn Collection, University of Pennsylvania and Pennsylvania Historical and Museum Commission.*

notion of a total environment. Both believed that the isolated and largely metal swings, slides, and seesaws that populated New York City's playgrounds, many left over from Robert Moses's time as parks commissioner (1934–1960), were limiting children's actions. Each designed playgrounds that linked children's activities, both horizontally and vertically, so that every space would be filled with things to do. Their sensitive and artistic conclusions showed that kids could be physically challenged and, given the right situation, execute complex play.

Their designs were complicated assemblages that indicated faith in children's ability to exercise sound judgments or, at least, to take limited risks and learn from their mistakes. Friedberg and Dattner each created playgrounds with a neutral, uncolored palette. Many of their designs interlinked stone mounds and wood frames. To a young population that had grown up with metal equipment, the introduction of wood and stone must have seemed a revelation. These play areas sat on sand that became both an inexpensive safety surface and a dynamic place to play.

An extant and excellent example of Dattner's work is the Adventure Playground (1966) in Central Park. He graciously cites the Kahn-Noguchi playground as his source (as does Carve in Amsterdam, when they note the same inspiration for their playhill at Billie Holiday Park in The Hague. See 1.2). Modified since its inception, Dattner's Adventure Playground still illustrates how children could clamber their way up stone pyramids, access a

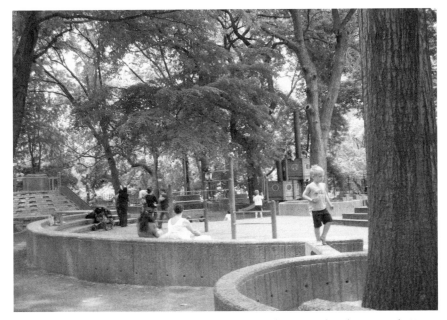

FIGURE 1.3 | *Richard Dattner, Adventure Playground in Central Park, New York City, 1966 (renovated 1997). The serpentine walls provide both climbing surfaces and backs for the tiered seating. The truncated stone pyramid, at left, allows for climbing and stored "loose parts" when the playground first opened. Author's photograph, 2009.*

tree house, hide in a series of tunnels, or play in a water channel. The low, concrete serpentine wall remains especially winning because it charmingly hugs the play space while providing an interesting structure for climbing, running, or balancing.[79]

Kahn and Noguchi were not the only influences on Dattner and Friedberg. Both young men admired and had met Lady Allen of Hurtwood, who later returned their admiration by publishing their projects in her 1968 book *Planning for Play*. Having seen that children in London could play amid the ruins left in the wake of the German Blitz, and familiar with the playgrounds that C. Th. Sørensen created from leftover household and building scraps in Denmark during the war, Lady Allen crusaded for the introduction of adventure play to Britain. She was very successful in seeing many adventure playgrounds come to fruition. These were sites in which children, under the watchful but noninterfering eye of a play worker, could use tools and "junk" in order to construct their own environments. Donne Buck, a New Zealander who began working at London's Notting Hill Adventure Playground shortly after it opened in 1960, has eloquently summed up the impact: "Children whose lives are otherwise circumscribed by age, disability, religion, ethnic origin, poverty, social strife etc. etc. can come together on an adventure playground from pre-school and find their own level amongst the mix of others in ways that they cannot anywhere else in their lives."[80] Play workers sometimes built semipermanent towers in order to maximize space and keep the oldest, most rambunctious kids working away from the smallest ones. These were an early armature, too. Donne Buck remembers building a high, triangular fifteen-foot tower. It was a strategy to refocus the energy of some unruly teens.[81] Buck's important message is that the older children were not evicted; they were given more interesting spaces to control.

The idea of malleable "loose parts" on the playground emerged from the leftover lumber, household materials, or junk that was available — effectively, the "equipment" of adventure playgrounds.[82] Not surprisingly, Dattner and Friedberg found ways to incorporate loose parts into their designs. Dattner, in particular, designed interlocking building vertical pieces for his own Adventure Playground (whose name echoed the European examples) in Central Park and provided storage for them within his stone pyramids. Dattner was effectively creating the foundation for energetic free play. Friedberg believed that urban playgrounds should be part of an intergenerational arrangement, and he sought a way to replicate the unexpected consequences children could experience in rural nature. His 1960s trailblazing work, an entire ensemble for the New York City Housing Authority's Riis Houses (Pomerance and Breines, 1949), has been altered beyond recognition. This was a twist and up-to-date abstraction of an earlier tradition, the re-creation of nature for an urban audience. New York's Central Park and San Francisco's Golden Gate Park had been early conveyors of that belief. The Adventure Playgrounds in England also had "landscape mounds" and green areas for digging soil and planting a garden.[83]

Although they look more refined than the rough, messy British or Scandinavian adventure playgrounds, the Dattner and Friedberg examples captured their spirit. Friedberg's and Dattner's self-contained playgrounds allowed children to be independent. Whether they came alone or with a caretaker kids dominated the scene, with adults remaining in the background. The adults formed their own social networks; so did the children. Anyone who thinks that Dattner and Friedberg had an overly romantic vision of adventure play should watch the initial installment of Michael Apted's Seven Up series. Apted first began to interview seven-year-olds from diverse backgrounds in 1964.[84] He has returned to the same people every seven years and issued a movie update after each encounter. He concluded his inaugural segment—which mixed children from elite and educated backgrounds with those from much more humble surroundings—with a trip for the children to meet each other in London. The children mixed together at a party; they also spent time together on an Adventure Playground. The producers saw the playground as a place where such a disparate population could find common activities. The kids show that the space—almost two decades after the concept emerged in the UK—encouraged physical activity, moving, and building objects, and the freedom to alter the environment.

The decline in American playground design has been apparent since the 1980s. Even in 1980 there were reports that traditional equipment was too safe and children were avoiding it.[85] It is disheartening that today's ubiquitous standardized equipment, called "post and deck" or "post and platform," which keeps the linkages but has oversimplified everything else, is a bastardized version of Dattner's and Friedberg's accomplishments. A small number of corporations now make American playground equipment, most of which is identical. The distinctions are often only in the colors—which, since the availability of inexpensive powder coating on metal in the 1980s, has created bizarre and lurid color possibilities; these odd hues have further cheapened the look of the post and deck designs. Our general societal concern for safety, the advent of the national safety guidelines, and the ongoing threat of litigation against schools and municipalities have all contributed to the success of manufactured equipment and its role as the defining element in the American playground.

Playgrounds Reflect Cultures

Playgrounds reflect a society's values and attitudes. Editors of a European journal make a distinction between "collectivist" Scandinavia, where the ethos is to support and aid each other, and the "individualist" mode, where each person watches out for himself (and presumably his chance of being sued). Setting up a dichotomy between collective and individualist societies does help to explain why many examples of the best playgrounds, the ones that will appear in the following chapters, exist in either Scandinavia or Northern Europe. In even broader terms, a "collective response," which has deep societal support, has the luxury to consider the greater good; an "individualistic response," in contrast, is self-protective, accommodates no risk, and shelters "surplus safety"—safety that exceeds what is reasonably necessary.[86] Nordic peoples or Northern Europeans emphasize life skills and socialization on the playground. These tools are essential for a collective point of view; public space becomes a training ground for social inter-action. Nordic countries, therefore, invest in public experiences and only begin to teach academics when children reach the age of seven.[87] Compare that situation to the English-speaking world, especially the United States and Australia, which has kept its individualistic focus and succumbed to an early education prototype that values content and testing over socialization or communal understanding. There is limited concern for play and play-grounds as part of an overall integrated experience.

Collectivist versus individualist thinking goes beyond educational issues. It extends to a sense of common responsibility. In Sweden, for example, the emphasis is on all citizens being responsible for all the children.[88] This collective view reassures parents that an adult is always watching their children; it also comforts kids by letting them know that they are being monitored for anything that is too outrageous. In such a trusting atmo-sphere, parents feel they can encourage their children to be self-reliant. The editors of one journal summed it up by asking "Should the dominant image of the child be one of vulnerability or competence"?[89] Does the child need protection or independence?

The United States presents a striking contrast to collectivist thinking. Ironically, our individualism may have nurtured dependency. Sociologist Claude S. Fischer uses the frame of "voluntarism" as the "central feature of American culture and character." Fischer defines voluntarism as belief and behavior "as if each person is a sovereign individual: unique, independent, self-reliant, self-governing, and ultimately self-responsible."[90] He concludes that American individualism is "coupled with intense, freely given fellow-ship—group belonging by voluntary contract or covenant" in which there has to be a balance between deep commitment for good of the group and in-dependence.[91] In Fischer's assessment, self-reliance and self-responsibility are protective; we have strong—but not necessarily unbreakable—loyalties to national institutions; our defining instincts are self-sustaining. Historian Paula Fass has called this the "privatization of responsibility."[92] This alle-giance to self-protection helps to explain why we have spent years debating national health insurance, whereas European countries have long had uni-versal coverage. To us, health care is an entitlement, a gift; to them, it is the means that keep a society functioning by lessening public health threats.

These distinctions are evident in how national guidelines for play-grounds have different emphases. When we contrast the 2008 voluntary European Playground Equipment Standards with the American CPSC's guidelines from the same year, we see that the Europeans accept risk and recognize the possibility of injury; Americans try to control all vulnerability. They offer their children latitude; we offer our kids the promise of individual total protection. In both instances, the guidelines have to accommodate wide regional and cultural distinctions within their respective political boundaries. The European standards note:

> Respecting the characteristics of children's play and the way children benefit from playing on the playground with regard to development, children need to learn to cope with risk and this may lead to bumps and bruises and even occasionally a broken limb. The aim of this standard is first and foremost to prevent accidents with a disabling or fatal consequence, and secondly to lessen serious consequences caused by the occasional mishap that inevitably will occur in children's pursuit of expanding their level of competence, be it socially, intellectually or physically.[93]

The u.s. cpsc begins its guidelines by lumping together all negative outcomes, all of which it is committed to reducing: "In recent years, it is estimated that there were more than 200,000 injuries annually on public playgrounds across the country that required emergency room treatment. By following the recommended guidelines in this handbook, you and your community can create a safer playground environment for all children and contribute to the reduction of playground-related deaths and injuries."[94]

Japan is also home to some superb playgrounds, and that country gives its own spin to a "collective" spirit.[95] Japan's concept of *Uchi* (inside) starts at immediate family, expands to school, and extends outward to all of Japan (or to all Japanese people). When children start school, they are all equal and part of a new *Uchi*; they are expected to cooperate with each other. The school then expands the "cocoon" of the clan or the home into a wider, more diverse support system. Shared responsibility means that there is a mutual help and mutual trust system and concern for people younger than themselves. This attitude fits with a goal of creating harmony and balance in society. Under those conditions, it makes sense that three-year-olds (provided they don't live near busy streets) will often play outside their houses by themselves. Even kindergartners are expected to walk to a fixed spot where they meet other children and walk together to class. Part of the first grade curriculum in Tokyo (albeit an exceptionally safe city) is learning to get to school alone, a journey that might include crossing streets or riding a subway or bus.[96] In the less dense areas of the city, in the wards where there are no sidewalks, there is further evidence of how the Japanese orchestrate a civil society: children learn to be wary of cars and cars are careful of pedestrians, so that each group shows deference to the other and learns how to navigate shared space.[97]

We cannot change our culture. But acceptance of national character does not give us license to tolerate mediocre public space or isolated places for children that are absurdly boring and financially wasteful. Perhaps we can begin to demand more successful outcomes, especially in urban areas, if we know what is possible and see how other countries are using open areas to help their children grow. Knowing what is available in other societies should be a catalyst for us; perhaps we can try to overcome our ingrained instincts and emulate useful attitudes and the designs they produce.

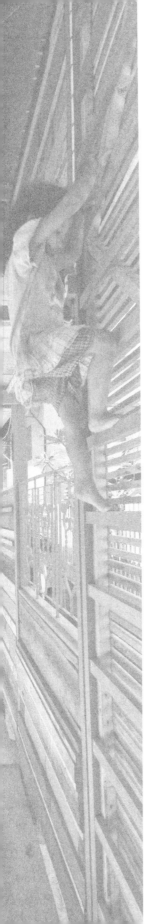

Risk and Independence

RISK, FAILURE, AND MASTERY are a tight trio. They are interconnected. This chapter concentrates on the value of risk taking for child development. It considers projects that are exemplary for encouraging those traits. The following chapter continues the theme by examining sites that are particularly effective at encouraging children to master a given situation after first encountering difficulty or failure. Taken together, these chapters indicate the scope of risk independence, failure, success.

Defining Risk

The notion of risk taking is a hard sell, particularly in America. For governmental agencies, risk taking ignites fear of litigation; for parents, it stimulates deep concern for the well-being of their children. It is an especially problematic concept to accept when our culture works assiduously to eliminate it. When we think about taking risks, we conjure up images of children walking on unprotected rooftops or chasing a ball into a road with fast-moving traffic. Those activities are actually hazards, not risks. We need to appreciate how risks and hazards differ. Risk means a situation with an unclear outcome; nothing is predetermined.[1] Making choices may be part of risk taking.[2] Hazards, which are never acceptable, also have unclear conclusions but harbor the possibility of life-threatening dangers.[3] Risk, which accepts the possibility of minor injuries, can be a valuable part of every childhood experience.

Mike Shooter, former president of the Royal College of Psychiatrists, writes: "Children and adolescents must naturally take risks as they explore the physical world and its emotional relationships. Parents who overprotect children may cause just as much harm as those who neglect them. Sheltered from all experience of risk, such children may be unable to cope when they meet it outside the family home. Others may rebel in dangerous ways against the web their parents weave around them. In other words, an optimum amount of risk is a healthy part of growing up."[4] Shooter's message validates the conclusion that Lady Allen reached almost a half-century earlier: "It is often difficult to permit children to take risks, but over-concern prevents them from growing up."[5]

The encouraging message, especially for parents, is that risk is not as harrowing as we might imagine. Ellen Beate Hansen Sandseter, who teaches psychology at Queen Maud University College of Early Childhood Education in Trondheim, Norway, is a leading scholar of risk.[6] In the broadest terms, she defines risky play, which usually occurs outdoors, as "thrilling and exciting forms of play that involve a risk of physical injury."[7] The odds are in favor of most kids escaping injury, since "a relatively small proportion of children tend to account for a large proportion of injuries."[8] She identifies the characteristics of risky play as achieving fast speeds; going to great heights; being able to vanish or get lost; using potentially harmful tools; playing near dangerous areas; and rough-and-tumble play (see chapter 6 for more information on rough-and-tumble, R&T).[9]

These risky attributes, none of which have a predetermined conclusion, look less terrifying to adults when we see that they can mean running down steep slopes, biking at high speeds, jumping from high places, sliding high and fast, and hiding. Some parents may not be as pleased to recognize some of the other activities that fit the bill: swinging, especially if it incorporates jumping off in midflight; playing on cliffs that could be six to nine feet above the ground; standing at or near a fire pit; whittling with a knife, or constructing with hammer, nails, or saws.[10] As Sandseter points out, children negotiate their way between truly horrifying activities and the ones that are just scary;[11] when they reach their own sense of equilibrium, they express delight by laughing, shouting, smiling, screaming, and yelling.[12] There is glee in having an experience for which there is not a single route or a known conclusion.

Sandseter and a colleague speculate (their work is in the very early stages of investigation) that risk taking may serve an evolutionary necessity. They believe that very young children have real fears. These are the biological weapons that prevent them from trying things at which they are not developmentally ready to succeed. But if kids have a chance to slowly overcome those fears (water, darkness, heights), they end up learning skills at an appropriate age. Risk taking benefits maturation. Children who are removed from these beneficial risks might face increased neurotic and pathological fears as they get older. Anxious children who are overprotected might become more anxious because they have not had a chance to confront and control their fears.[13]

Neuroscientists look at the situation a little differently; they believe that children's risk taking may be a developmental factor that "tests boundaries and establishes what is safe and what is dangerous."[14] Kids have to take chances, to constantly experience risks, if they are going to adapt to the world around them. We can tell from the gleeful yelling and screaming that they are finding it pleasurable. Here, too, neuroscientists view enjoyment in terms of continuing our existence by noting that "we are wired to like activities that are helpful for our survival."[15] It becomes a purposeful cycle: we test our capacity to try things by taking risks; we find pleasure in it; we take more risks, and so on. As a plus, pleasurable activity increases dopamine (the transmitter related to award expectation) and decreases stress hormones.[16]

Assessing and managing risk is another aspect of engaging with it.[17] The key to successful risk taking is being able to adapt its lessons to unexpected situations in the future.[18] Helen Little, at the Institute of Early Childhood of Macquarie University in Sydney, suggests, "The ability to assess potentially risky situations and avoid excessive risks is an important life skill and one which constantly changes during childhood in response to developing abilities and knowledge in different contexts."[19] We don't give kids enough credit for this; scientists know they withdraw when they sense that fear is overwhelming.[20] When they become uncomfortable with what they are doing, they stop doing it.[21]

Taking risks, assessing dangers, and managing potential consequences do not have to be petrifying. While fatalities are never acceptable, we have to ask if it is in everyone's best interest for Americans to try to eliminate all playground risks and injuries. We need to applaud and encourage the few municipalities that are willing to buck the national trend to make playgrounds as safe as possible. We must look abroad and see the exciting ways that designers are folding risk into playground design without creating hazards. We have a good deal to learn from their examples.

Simple Solutions: Stones, Tools, See-Saws

Sometimes unpretentious designs can elicit the most successful risk taking, whereby even toddlers can take part in a self-determined "risk-management exercise."[22] A serene seventeen-acre public park and arboretum in Princeton, New Jersey, is an unlikely site for risky activity. Just a few blocks away from the New Jersey governor's mansion, Marquand Park has low, rustic, split-rail fences where it abuts the streets. The descendants of Alan Marquand, an eminent art historian in Princeton University's Depart-

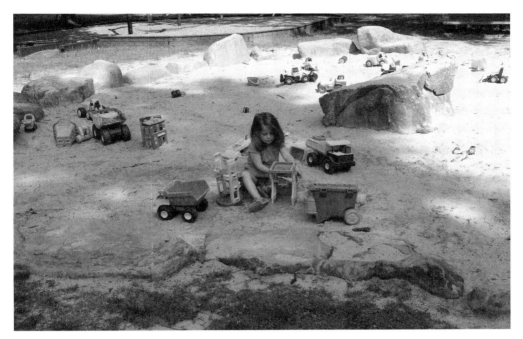

FIGURE 2.1 | *Sand Pit (1980s), Marquand Park, Princeton, New Jersey. Until early 2013, the perimeter was composed entirely of rough stones; several have been removed and replaced by flatter ones to allow "easier" access. Photograph by Robert S. Solomon, 2013.*

ment of Art and Archeology, established this green area of unusual trees and extensive pathways in 1953; the municipality has maintained it pristinely ever since.[23]

The park's sandpit, a rarity on many playgrounds, shows how it is possible to introduce risk into the world of a two-year-old. This circular pit is quite large; there is no fencing to cordon it off from the rest of the park or the nearby parking lot. Low boulders (slightly altered in 2013) ring the exterior and an additional hefty rock, which poses challenges for tiny climbers, sits in the center of the pit. These local stones, each handpicked by Marquand's granddaughter Elinor Forseyth at a nearby quarry, have a rugged aesthetic appeal.[24] It is instantly clear that these are not the "faux rocks" that come from today's catalogs. The sand here is filled with broken toys that children leave. These relics seem to indicate that kids return regularly, or that all the participants have a need for "loose parts" and for manipulating their environment.

The real significance of this sand area becomes evident to anyone spending some time there. School-age kids run or jump from rock to rock. The rocks are close together but still require good balance and careful judgment.

It is not unusual to see a toddler arrive with a pail and shovel. In one instance in 2010, a two-year-old girl (let's call her "Maggie") arrived holding one of these brand-new implements in each hand. She was animated and excited to be there. Maggie stopped short and paused when she reached the rocks. She took a quick glance around; for a split second she was not sure how to enter the pit; then she threw her pail and shovel into the sand. Unencumbered and with free hands, she lowered herself onto the rocks and into the sand. It was breathtaking to watch. This small child had made an assessment; she realized she couldn't surmount the rocks while her hands were occupied. She recognized a danger; she assessed the risk and figured out how to manage it. In the end, she used reasoning and planning to solve what, for her, was at first a daunting problem. Sandseter's message that risk is normal, necessary, and should not be taken away from children's daily lives plays out at the sand and rock pit.[25] Maggie certainly would have had a less memorable encounter if there had been an ordinary sandbox and someone had just lifted her into it.

It is heartening that Princeton has used the Marquand Park sandpit as a model for a sand area in the recent renovation of its Harrison Street Park. This renovation, in a different part of town, had several false starts and tentative schemes. Ultimately, Edgewater Design created a smaller version of the Marquand Park sandpit. The designers called for a circular sand area with a natural rock perimeter. This time, the rock came from a building project. The Islamic Society of Central New Jersey, in nearby Monmouth Junction, was digging to build a retention basin; Princeton municipality was able to secure the excavated rocks and repurpose them. This sustainable choice saved the town a significant amount of money; the cost to transport and position the stone was less than $5,000. It was a modest price (the entry-level commercial 16 x 16 sandbox is at least $6,000 prior to installation), will never deteriorate, and can accommodate many children.

While it's one thing to laud an unusual sandbox, it might be something else to encourage parents to let young children use sharp, potentially dangerous tools. Most American adults shudder when they consider their children using saws and knives. But here, too, there are ways to introduce risky play with tools without resorting to exotic measures. Adventure playgrounds, such as those advocated by Lady Allen of Hurtwood in Britain, have long offered kids the opportunity to play with objects that might, in other settings, be deemed dangerous. These facilities give children the chance to use knives, saws, and paint to construct their own play worlds.

Adventure playgrounds, which have a distinguished history in the United

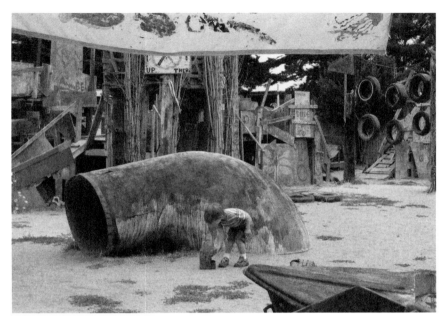

FIGURE 2.2 | *Adventure Playground, Berkeley, California. This playground,*
which has operated continuously since 1979, has not had any life-altering injuries.
Author's photograph, 2009.

Kingdom and are currently flourishing in Japan, have never gained a strong
following in America. The Adventure Playground in Berkeley, California, is
the only one in the United States that is permanent and functioning year-
round. It began in the 1970s, has been running continuously ever since,
and has never had a serious injury.[26] The playground appears to be more
risky than it really is; the illusion of danger is powerful for kids. They get to
prove that they can evaluate tools, carefully use them, and build fantastical
assemblages.

The Berkeley Adventure Playground came about by chance. In 1978,
the city had an enterprise zone on its waterfront, including a marina and
restaurant, but not many visitors. The city, hearing that the Adventure
Playground Association was sponsoring a workshop, sent a young parks department employee, Patty Donald, to the event. Several communities sent
delegates, but Berkeley was the only one to follow through, largely because
there was a political will to create something. The concept of adventure
play outlined at the workshop was seductive: the only ongoing costs would
be staffing and maintenance; the start-up money for materials and fencing
would be minimal. Nothing would be static: the park could accept continuing contributions of "junk" and, if the structures built by the children grew

too large or too permanent, the staff could take them down and children could rebuild them over successive years.

Donald and her assistants were clever in how they introduced the Adventure Playground, sited in a former parking lot, to the community. During the first years, they paid to transport children from local recreation centers to the site. Donald, who had grown up in Berkeley, reached out to everyone she knew. She traded a case of beer for the transportation of redundant telephone poles. She prevailed on contractors to donate leftover wood. Slowly, she added more tools and more materials until she made it a fascinating site, a place that she says now is "loved to death" by more than eighty thousand kid visits each year.

The Berkeley playground, which offers the same opportunities today that it did when it opened, continues to put tools (especially saws) into the hands of young children. Children get to use hammers and nails, too. They do not do so unattended; they receive instruction on the proper way to handle dangerous implements and must abide by clear rules. Children have to collect a certain number of rusty nails or dangerous splinters to "earn" their tools. With recent donations of old pianos and harps, the kids have to be ready to handle unusual objects. They get to attempt things that they have not tried before, and for which there is no predetermined conclusion. There is a social aspect, too. When using such dangerous tools as knives, children talk to each other because they continually verbalize (and reassure themselves) how important it is to use the tools correctly.[27]

The Adventure Playground continues, but Donald increasingly sees kids who come to the park unprepared to walk on uneven ground or unsure of how to climb up or down a hill. She is sad to see this but perseveres, hoping to acclimate kids to a taste of the world. How funny, then, that children have used a board and some logs to create a seesaw from scraps of wood found at the Adventure Playground, even though a real fulcrum seesaw is as hard to find on an American playground as a knife or saw. Americans have forsaken it. Afraid of litigation, manufacturers have reduced the seesaw to a long, thin artificial log with a small spring at the center. The "totter" has almost no mobility. An alternative design includes an enclosed seat so that kids can't fall. Oddly, the CPSC guidelines allow for something more adventuresome, a full-fledged, high, potentially terrorizing model. The old-fashioned kind that could give kids a thrill and a scare (can you trust your companion not to dump you?) fits within the federal guidelines, provided that a half-tire is inserted in the ground as proper cushioning.

Rare in America, the traditional seesaw is not uncommon in Europe, where it provides a sense of risk for teens and even younger children (see figure c.3). Designers there do not hesitate to create their own versions, often with wood, so that kids can raise each other up and even dump each other off. It is a shame that Americans have jettisoned an inexpensive way to offer sanctioned risk to their offspring.

Hiding In Plain Sight

In Scandinavia, where there is an old adage that says, "There is no such thing as cold weather, only children who are not dressed properly," outdoor facilities for kids are heavily used and welcome throughout the year. The Norwegian Framework Plan for the Content and Task of Kindergartens (Kunnskapsdepartementet, 2006) reinforces outdoor play as the central element in the early lives of children. There is general understanding that play, especially outdoor play, is the "content" and the "task" referred to in the title; the underlying belief is that play, social interaction, and experiential exploration will enhance social and cognitive development because everything is open-ended.[28] Kids will "learn risk mastery."[29] Vygotsky's principles are thriving in this setting, which emphasizes social and contextual cooperation.[30]

The Framework Plan, part of a broader reform effort to provide universal childcare (when combined with private daycares) for children from birth to age six in a country where there is no unemployment, spawned many new facilities.[31] Called "kindergartens," these facilities have had opportunities to devise innovative ways to consider the playground.

Marit Justine Haugen and Dan Zohar are architects (Haugen/Zohar) in Oslo who designed a playground addition intended for children ages two to five, for whom hiding is the risky charm of being outdoors. Their cube for Breidablikk Kindergarten in Trondheim is in a schoolyard,[32] one that is open twenty-four hours a day so that families can gravitate toward it whenever they wish. The twelve-square-meter cube is built from preindustrial waste — specifically, open-cell xp foam (recycled from the automotive and shoe industries) that would have been placed in a landfill or burned if it had not been repurposed. The architects thermally bonded the waste chips, glued compressed strips of it to form a solid block, and then used a water jet cutter to hollow it out. At 1.5 tons, the structure is both stable and self-draining.

The result is a dignified, haunting cube that morphs into a "Cave." The speckle-colored exterior is dark but eye-catching. The architects "carved" several exterior niches where children can place their found "treasures."

Unexpected activity takes place inside. The architects, who found inspiration in natural caves in Norway, provide spaces "to hide, climb, explore and lose yourself within a secretive, spooky space."[33] Kids (the cube can hold thirty-six inside, plus one adult) can entertain themselves in a small entry space that gets light from an oculus at the top. From the entrance "room," they see what appears to be a dark tunnel on a slightly upward-tilting grade. It is confining, scary, and slippery; in winter, it is icy. Kids can help each other slither up and slide down. If they are able to make their way up higher, they come to a small room. Another passage leads to an even higher space. Haugen/Zohar thought carefully about how best to create a series of spatially expanding and contracting experiences for the kids who want to reach the "peak." Light, sunlight, and darkness all alter the effects. These rooms are kid-size; the children have to navigate with peers or go alone. In an emergency a teacher could come in, but difficult access ensures that this is truly a zone where kids are "lost." The space is so secretive and soundproof that children who are inside cannot hear their parents when they come at pickup time.

The Cave shows that there are adults who have an inherent trust in kids and their ability to conduct themselves carefully, removed from the adult world; it also demonstrates that beautifying the environment is an accept-

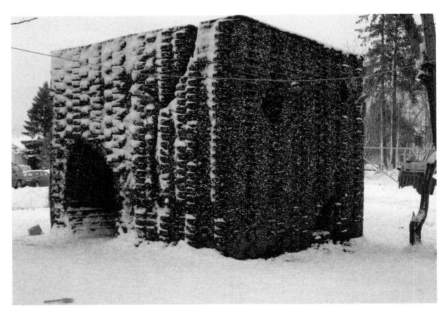

FIGURE 2.3 | *Haugen/Zohar Arkitekter, Cave at Breidablikk Kindergarten in Trondheim, Norway, 2012.* The Architectural Review *chose this for an award in its 2011 AR+D Emerging Architecture program. Author's photograph, 2012.*

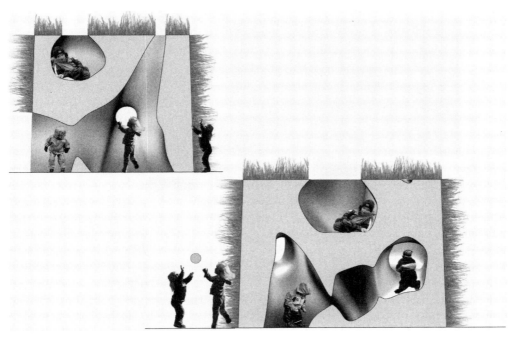

FIGURE 2.4 | *Haugen/Zohar Arkitekter, sections of Cave at Breidablikk Kindergarten in Trondheim, Norway, 2012. The architects created a sophisticated sequence of compressed and open spaces that children experience in their climb to the top. Courtesy of Haugen/Zohar Arkitekter.*

able part of healthy living. This play space has architectural and artistic integrity, having been a runner-up for the 2011 AR+D Awards for Emerging Architecture. It can be valued, also, as a piece of art. Haugen/Zohar won this commission (which cost a relatively small amount, about $60,000, in a country where an ordinary sandwich and coffee can run $30) through a local Percent for Art program. The award further confirms that outdoor material spaces for children are compatible with high aspirations for artwork and have the ability to enhance surroundings.

The Percent for Art Initiative, as outlined in Trondheim's master plan for 2001 to 2012, makes explicit the connection between art and enriched living: "A good urban environment has as its prerequisite focus on art and culture, architecture and infrastructure based on a holistic view of people. Our challenge is to provide art and culture with an overall role in the development of urban society as a whole." Accordingly, the city sets aside 1.25 percent of its capital budget for art projects, leaving open the amount that can be allocated to each venue. The program has been particularly active in providing art, including sophisticated lighting systems for the short winter days, for the new kindergarten buildings.[34] Artists, who must pledge not to replicate the pieces they provide for the program, get the chance to adapt art to everyday routines. Most significantly, the program demonstrates how a society can use art to support kids' activities, including climbing and hiding, as a means to improve life in the city and, by establishing unique pieces, forge a sense of identity and place.

In Tokyo, kids can do a different kind of disappearing by playing in dense fog. It, too, is a work of art. Fog Forest (also called "misty forest") was a collaboration of architect Atsushi Kitagawara and artist Fujiko Nakaya. Nakaya had been creating fog sculptures for more than two decades; Kitagawara was just starting his architecture practice (he is now known internationally and has an office in Berlin in addition to Tokyo) when the two received this commission in the early 1990s. Fog Forest is in Showa Kinen, a national park within Tokyo. Under the aegis of the Ministry of Land Infrastructure and Transport, this park is a large (more than four-hundred-acre) varied space on the site of a former air base in Tachikawa district. Planned in the late 1970s to mark the fiftieth anniversary of Emperor Hirohito's reign, the park has been opened in phases since 1983. The children's area of the park has several distinct sites, any of which could stand independently as a unique playground.

The Fog Forest captivates both children and adults. Twice an hour, a thick mist envelops the site, particularly a deep, square, man-made "funnel-formed lake." The entire area is enclosed in the impenetrable fog. Atmospheric conditions determine where the fog will sit and for how long. Kids can easily wander around and even jump on low truncated pyramids of closely clipped grass ("lawn mounds") that surround the lake on all sides but are not distributed uniformly. Children can hide there until the fog disperses. When the fog has gone, all people tend to gather around the empty lake, almost unsure of what they have just witnessed. They have been part of a powerful ephemeral event that shrouded them and then dissipated. Visitors seem to long for it to occur again, possibly hoping that they can capture the fog on their next try. Architect Kitagawara is actually displeased that a rail surrounds the "fog pond." He had wanted people to descent into it, and believes the current handrail destroys the mystery and risk — not being able to see anything — that he had wanted to create.[35]

For children, there is special pleasure in feeling removed, even lost, and then recovering the ground. It is unclear how much they grasp the significance of the grass mounds, meant to be climbable and reflective of grave mounds. Kitagawara wanted to invoke Japanese reverence for nature and

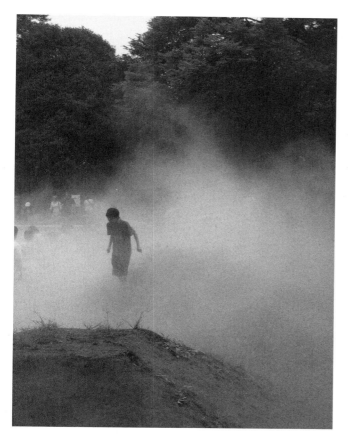

FIGURE 2.5

*Atsushi Kitagawara and
Fujiko Nakaya, Fog Forest at
Showa Kinen Park, Tokyo, 1992.
Author's photograph, 2006.*

the continuing cycle of life and death. The experience is totally different from the light sprays for cooling off that are sometimes found in American urban playgrounds. This Japanese play spot, which is more than twenty years old, continues to capture a universal need to hide and be away from everyone nearby.[36]

Climbing High and Running Fast

BASE (Bien Aménager Son Environnement/Build a Super Environment) is a landscape architecture firm in France. The principals, Franck Poirier, Bertrand Vignal, and Clément Willemin, met when they were students at the Versailles National School of Landscape Architecture and from which they graduated in 2000. From their first association, they made a conscious decision to design only public spaces or spaces for nonprofit endeavors.[37] They have since expanded into a team of more than twenty-five landscape designers, architects, and engineers with offices in Paris, Lyon, and Bordeaux.

Playgrounds occupy a central place in their philosophy. Willemin articulates the firm's view: "A playground is the best thing that can be done for a district; it provides something distinctive. Playgrounds are objects of identification and qualification of which the residents can be proud."[38] This view held them in good stead when Paris sought a designer to replace an old playground in Belleville Park, at the second-highest elevation in the city.

Before the city of Paris committed to a plan and a design firm, it conducted a one-year study to see what parents in the neighborhood wanted. CODEJ (*le Comité pour la Développement d'Espaces pour le Jeu*), working on behalf of the city, carried out workshops. Among other things, CODEJ asked parents to rank values such as security, imagination, and risk. Simultaneously, the city asked the seven competing design teams to enunciate their firms' core values. BASE was a perfect match for the community: both had put risk at the top of their lists. The parents in this neighborhood, made up largely of immigrants from Arabic-speaking countries and China, asked for something that would embody the challenging landscapes amid which they had grown up; they did not want a piece of plastic equipment, but they did request a place where eight- to twelve-year-olds would come often and be safe by themselves.

The BASE-designed playground in Belleville Park, which retains the footprint and entrances of the wooden structure from the 1970s (closed in 2000) it replaced, appears at first glance to be perilous. Made of concrete and wood, it rises at a 30-degree angle over a thirty-six-foot elevation. Nestled in a corner of the park, the playground has a low unobtrusive fence to keep the smallest tots away. Like an Adventure Playground, it offers challenges while remaining quite safe. Since the playground's completion in 2008, the sole major injury has been a cut above the eye that needed stitches; that child reportedly returned to the playground later in the day.[39] Unlike an Adventure Playground, the Belleville Park playground was an expensive proposition, costing more than $1.5 million (€1.1 million), but it is large (a thousand square meters) and accommodates hundreds of children at once. BASE deliberately minimized the number of seats for adults in order to ensure an atmosphere that cultivates self-reliance in kids.

At the bottom, kids can use ropes—or they could try crawling—to navigate up a concrete slope with changing planes. It's a training ground for learning that there are many different ways to achieve a goal. Like mountain climbing, one of the designers' inspirations, there is no single route to the next level. Once kids travel up far enough to reach the wooden section at the summit of this first level, they enter a dark overhang. There, they have

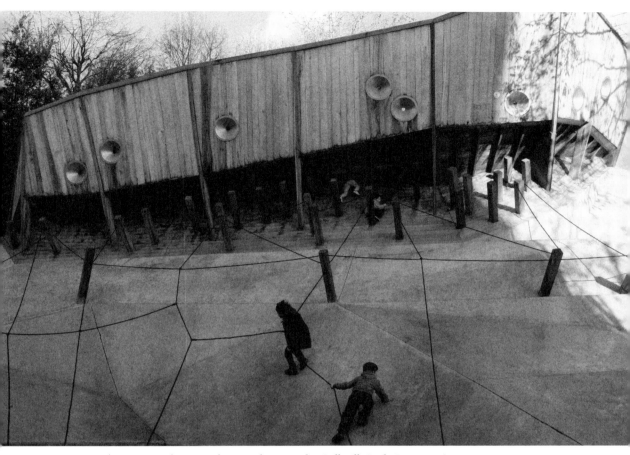

FIGURE 2.6 | *BASE Landscape Architects, playground in Belleville Park, Paris, 2008. This is the playground at its lowest point. Children use ropes to hoist themselves up to the enclosed area under the wood facing. Photograph by Robert S. Solomon, 2012. (Plate 1)*

to make choices; some paths will be dead ends. Eventually, some children will find an opening that will allow them to hoist themselves onto a second level terrace, at which point they encounter yet more choices: shifting wood planes, a wood climbing frame, nets, and stairs. As a unit, the wood structure provides many opportunities for climbing and balancing. If kids climb up to the third level, they reach another terrace. This one has a wood tower for them to climb; when they reach the top of that, they find high, level ground. BASE installed several Ping-Pong tables at this level. It quickly becomes apparent to those who use the playground that this is the place for adults who want to be nearby, but away from, the area where active play occurs. From here, children can either take a quick slide (two of the three slides are from the original play structure) or take a series of steps to the bottom of the playground, where the more intense activity resumes. Or they can exit directly to the street.

Children are constantly assessing and reassessing their journey to the top of the Belleville Park play space. Observing them, one sees what Sandseter has been pronouncing for several years: kids are adept at identifying their fears; they overcome them by regulating their own risky play.[40] They can quit on each of the terraces if the climb becomes too harrowing. BASE has made sure that children are constantly aware of choices, even if they can't predict the end results. Although the first level has a mazelike quality, in that children may come to a dead end, the playground offers varied ways to get to the top; kids choose the paths that suit them. There is no single route or path.

Another major park renovation, this time in Amsterdam, similarly pushes

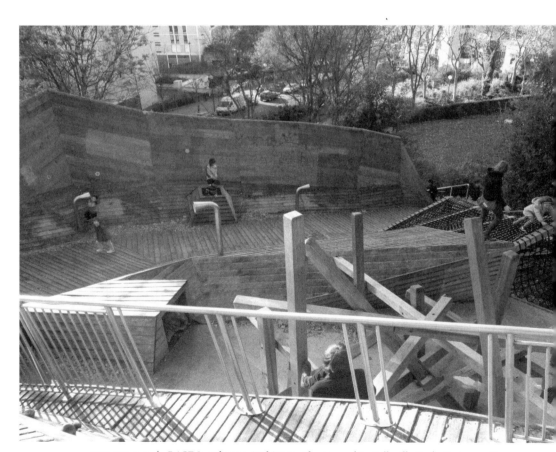

FIGURE 2.7 | *BASE Landscape Architects, playground in Belleville Park, Paris, 2008. This is the second higher level, where children reach the wooden terrace of the playground. Photograph by Robert S. Solomon, 2012. (Plate 2)*

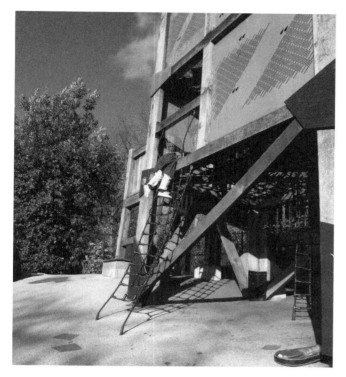

FIGURE 2.8

BASE Landscape Architects, playground in Belleville Park, Paris, 2008. This terrace leads to a climbing tower and eventually to an entrance at its highest point of the park. Photograph by Robert S. Solomon, 2012.

children to take risks, both real and perceptual, while climbing near a historic playground that Dutch architect Aldo van Eyck designed. Amsterdam once held an abundance of small, inexpensive playgrounds. Van Eyck designed more than seven hundred between 1945 and 1970. Taking advantage of small lots that had been abandoned or destroyed, or by commandeering traffic islands, van Eyck showed that playgrounds could be effective tools for community interaction in any available space.

Hallmarks of a van Eyck playground included a large sandbox, usually with a wide ledge at the top of its concrete wall, and a simple metal climbing dome, metal bars, or "stepping stones." A photo from the 1950s shows that the sandbox was the centerpiece of a packed public space. The sandbox could accommodate loads of kids; they could use the ledge for making sand pies. Their parents often used the ledge to sit, to view the children from a short distance, and to have a chat with other adults.

Van Eyck also demonstrated how to create a dense web of playgrounds within the urban environment so that children could move effortlessly from one to another. Local residents had to request a playground before van Eyck intervened. As Liane Lefaivre has shown, this was a grassroots, "bottom-up" request.[41]

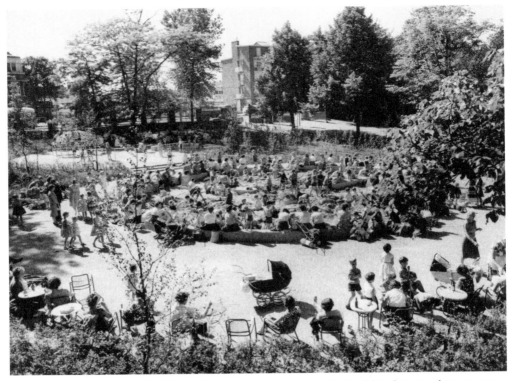

FIGURE 2.9 | *Aldo van Eyck, postwar playground in Vondel Park Amsterdam, ca. 1957. Van Eyck created a playground on two levels, a rarity for him. Courtesy of the Municipal Archives of Amsterdam.*

Unfortunately, many of the van Eyck playgrounds have disappeared over the years as commercial development has gobbled them up. There are still several along the interior edge of Amsterdam's late-nineteenth-century Vondel Park. Landscape architect Michael van Gessel took on the task of renovating and upgrading the park in 2001; in 2009, the design firm Carve came on board to handle the playgrounds. Carve, the same firm that designed the play hill in The Hague, is sensitive to history and has a deep respect for what van Eyck had accomplished. In many ways, Elger Blitz, Carve's cofounder, represents a possible model for young playground advocates. Perhaps because of his many years as a professional skateboarder, he accepts the notion of risk and strives to include it (or at least a feeling of risk) in diverse projects that come to his office.

For one of the van Eyck playgrounds in Vondel Park (the one pictured in Figure 2.9), Carve developed an upgrade that would make the space more appealing to older children while retaining the interest of younger ones.

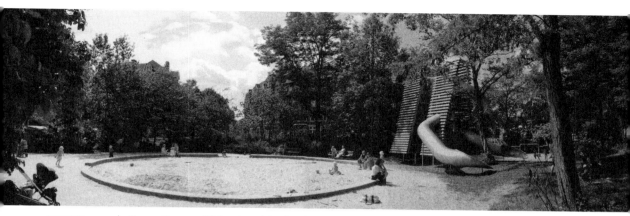

FIGURE 2.10 | *Carve. Tower addition (2010) in the playground designed by Aldo van Eyck at Vondel Park, Amsterdam. Van Eyck's sandpit is shown in the 1950s in the previous photograph. Courtesy of Carve.nl.*

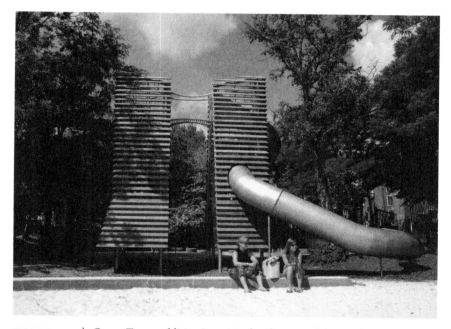

FIGURE 2.11 | *Carve. Tower addition (2010) in the playground designed by Aldo van Eyck at Vondel Park, Amsterdam. Courtesy of Carve.nl.*

This van Eyck playground is somewhat atypical in that the play equipment exists in two adjoining circular spaces, the smaller one of which was raised by a few low steps.

Carve chose to build only in the spot between the two play areas. In order to have the smallest intervention, they kept a discrete footprint by building high and retaining both sections of the van Eyck's play design. Carve has effectively created a vibrant vertical play element, their own version of van Eyck's reclaimed empty spaces.

Carve designed two wooden towers for the park.[42] The total cost was about €300,000 ($390,000). The wood-louvered slats that clad each tower are in homage to a nearby 1920s building that was built in the colonial style of Indonesia. The slats also protect kids from the overly watchful eyes of older folks. Children have several options through which to reach one of two slides that are connected to one of the towers. There is no need for safety surfacing, since the children can never fall more than a meter (three feet).

Kids decide, based on their tolerance of risk, how much challenge to handle. They could access one tower by moving up and across a series of platforms. The other tower is more daunting. Children have to find their way in and then hoist themselves along ropes and nets in order to ascend. If they fall, they have to start again. Eventually they can arrive at a bridge that is encapsulated in transparent mesh wire and is more than twenty feet off the ground. The effect, especially late in the day when the birds sing noisily, is similar to being in an aviary, although this time it is the children who are enclosed. They feel suspended — somewhat protected, somewhat exposed — from a very high position. From there, they can access a tall slide by which they can quickly reach the ground.

Another model for "moving high and fast" risky play can be found in the Maritime Youth House in Copenhagen (PLOT architects, a collaboration of Bjarke Ingels of BIG and Julien De Smedt of JDS 2004). This is a mixed-use site on Amager Island in Copenhagen harbor that stabilizes brownfields.[43] A key point of the original proposal was the removal of metallic waste from the site, a task that would have eaten up one-third of the budget. Since formal environmental remediation would have moved the soil only eight hundred meters away, PLOT wondered if there might be a better solution that would allow a larger portion of the budget for the other project goals: a youth outreach center and storage for the Sundby Sailing Club. PLOT chose to cover the tainted soil and invest the saved funds in building construction. The entire project was built for 1,450,000 Danish krone (about $270,000).

PLOT's innovative solution to the competing needs of the "sailors and the social workers" was to put the play space on the roof. Because all of the play area is located on top, the architects had plenty of room below to house the boats and create common rooms for social functions. The roof, with its distinctive undulating shape, became the noticeable feature. The designers

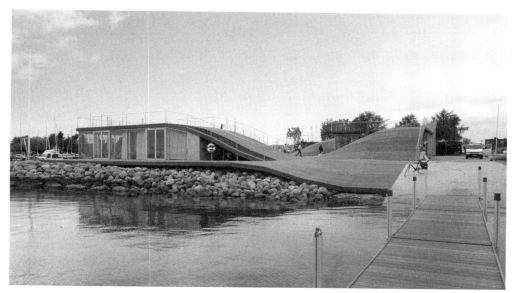

FIGURE 2.12 | *PLOT architects (a collaboration of Bjarke Ingels of BIG and Julien De Smedt of JDS), Maritime Youth House (2004), Copenhagen. Copyright and courtesy of PLOT=BIG+JDS.*

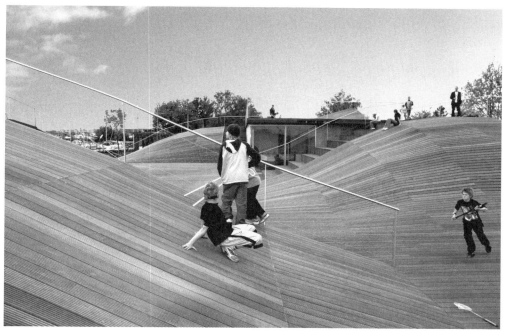

FIGURE 2.13 | *PLOT architects (a collaboration of Bjarke Ingels of BIG and Julien De Smedt of JDS), Maritime Youth House (2004), Copenhagen. Copyright and courtesy of PLOT=BIG+JDS.*

call it a "social carpet." They describe it as a play area, a "public landscape," a "wavy dune landscape materialized in wood." The deck includes steep areas, some up to 25 degrees, that allow children to experiment with traveling over elevated terrain.

Running on an open roof offers kids the chance to acquire speed, access height, and experience terrifying pleasure. In this particularly refined solution, the roof covers the shed but also dips down to the harbor. Since the roof was considered a public space, and not a promenade, building construction could directly abut the sea and forgo the usual eight-meter public promenade. Kids can build up some momentum and, if running down, have to be careful how to negotiate the place where the boat launch, sea, and roof meet. The steps and "slides" are particularly challenging in the winter, when they can be covered with snow. It is telling that the railing of metal and limited amount of wire mesh is minimal; it seems to be more of an outline for where the roof ends than a safety enclosure or fence.

The idea of siting a playground on a roof, of course, is not new. There is a long history of playgrounds on roofs, including their appearance on New York City tenements during the early twentieth century. The owner of the first Waldorf Astoria Hotel (site of the present Empire State Building) invited Playground Association of New York to bring "apparatus" to the rooftop in 1909. He was hoping to demonstrate how rooftops could be used for development of supervised playgrounds.[44] Even Le Corbusier's apartment complex in Marseille from the 1950s, Unité d'Habitation, had a play area on the flat top. Previous iterations were self-contained—although they might have had their own sense of displacement by being in the air—whereas this one in Copenhagen initiates the sense of real danger in running down so close to the sea.

Teens and the Lure of Electronic Games

While teens can gravitate to the roof of the Maritime Youth House or the playground in Belleville Park, they have few similar options in the United States. Contemporary American playgrounds don't hold or inspire older kids. One of two things happens as kids mature and tire of traditional post and deck equipment. They either use the equipment inappropriately, or they don't bother to use it at all. From around age eight, kids reinvent the old equipment to find the unexpected, creating dangers that exaggerate the risks that are missing from the playground experience. This is when they start to do truly terrifying things that are not always benign. They find a thrill, for instance, in using the top of equipment as a landing space for summersaults.[45] This type of behavior can—not surprisingly—lead to more severe injuries than would be produced through normal risk taking, although the number of injuries is still quite low.[46] When older children have exhausted the ways they can rework the equipment, they turn on each other by pushing and punching.

More and more, preteens avoid the playground altogether, choosing instead to spend time indoors, most likely sitting in front of some kind of screen. We all know that teens are hooked on games; they are discovering electronics at ever earlier ages, and it is hard to lure them away. Playground manufacturers, very aware of these trends, have confronted the problem in varying ways. One approach is to attach game imagery—such as, from the popular game Angry Birds—onto ordinary swings and slides. Other providers have attempted to tie the mechanics of games (bright lights, moving targets) to new equipment for adolescents, sometimes going so far as to include screens in their designs. The screens are hard to see in daylight, and the graphics usually have as much sophistication as an old Pac-Man display. What teen will go to the playground to play a game when he has better graphics at home on his computer or anywhere on his cell phone?

A different strategy, and one that has not been fully considered by playground equipment manufacturers, would be to embrace the essence of video games for what they do, not for how they appear. That strategy could provide exactly what's usually missing from parks and playgrounds. We should consider: What do games demand of users, and how could those demands be adapted into public space? Once we realize that games are meant to be exhilarating, risky, not always winnable, and requiring a great deal of practice, then we see that there is an overlap with the experiences that help children mature. There might even be strategies to adapt how teens use games to explore, show off, and interact in a fantasy world.[47]

Games create a sense of "being fully alive, focused, and engaged in every moment" as an "exhilarating and creative game accomplishment"; when played with others online, they create a sense of "power, heroic purpose, and community."[48] Jane McGonigal, in her engrossing book *Reality Is Broken*, maintains that humans desperately need to renew this sense of accomplishment, success, and total engagement. She notes that doing hard work gives us pleasure and is more satisfying than less demanding, possibly more passive activities. And all of these feelings of exhilaration can be derived from video games.[49]

Electronic games have even more similarities with successful play areas when we see that they might be immediately playable, be voluntary, have

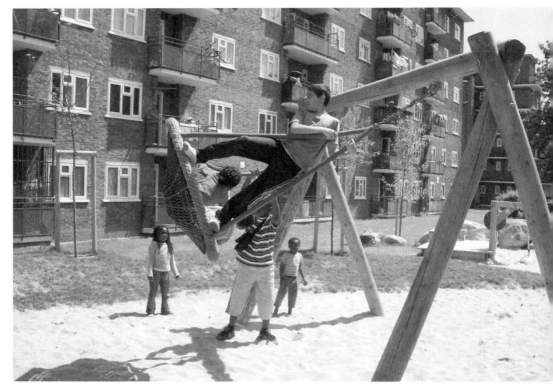

FIGURE 2.14 | *Teens often pile on and then soar high on bucket (also called "nest") swings. This one is at the Frampton Park housing estate in Hackney, London. Courtesy of Tim Gill (www.rethinkingchildhood.com).*

obstacles, have a sense of purpose (goals), and provide an immediate feedback system. In addition, McGonigal says that games are habit forming because they cause us to work to optimum ability; this pleasurable sensation is something psychologists call "flow." Indeed, "flow" may be more satisfying than actually winning. Good games are hard, and they produce a sense of accomplishment and optimism and a surge of continuing interest.[50]

Requirements for successful games appear complex and somewhat difficult to incorporate into physical reality, particularly public outdoor settings. Paradoxically, there are spaces that meet the same objectives, will attract teens, and don't cost a lot of money. Some of the best implements to accommodate the requirements are the most basic items that a manufacturer produces. We have already seen that simple solutions, such as irregular rocks lining a sandpit or an old fashioned seesaw, can provide manageable risks for young folks. It turns out that similarly uncomplicated solutions can entice older children.

Consider, for example, the large bucket swing, a staple of many playground equipment manufacturers. On one Barcelona street corner, teens fly out the door at the end of the school day and head for a small playground across the road. They scramble onto the oversize flat swing. First, they see how many can fit onto the saucer-shaped bucket. (Young folks are always attracted to the notion that more of them can fit into a space than should be humanely possible, as evidenced by crazes in the past for forcing each other into telephone booths or tiny cars.) Then, with one person left out, or through some ritual of their own devising, at least one person pushes while the others pump wildly. There is a clear feeling of exhilaration, accomplishment, and community as the group propels itself ever higher and higher. There is shared discovery of an ongoing process of swinging faster.

Architect Aase Eriksen, writing in the 1980s, recognized even then the "joy and terror of swinging high."[51] Even little children know that; the three- and four-year-old set head first to the swings. Architect Césare Peeren, doing some on-the-ground research for designing his own playground, took his eleven-year-old son to see more than a dozen facilities. They quickly concluded that every playground needs some sort of swing. The traditional flat swing is serviceable, but it is also possible, as Peeren has shown, to rely on an updated swing. In the 1970s, old tires found second lives in popular swings and climbing walls. Peeren (2012Architecten, now Superuse Studios) has used a swing that the Netherlands company Acacia Robinia sells. Their name implies the use of the hard robinia (black locust) tree, and, in fact, the swing includes a hexagonal frame made from stripped tree trunks. One swinging tire hangs suspended from each side of the frame. Kids can't swing far enough to bump into each other, but they can come close enough that there is a sensation of doing something dangerous (see figure 5.3).

Peeren's playground, and all the previous projects, illustrate how risk can be both useful and favorable. Another theme that runs through each of these endeavors is the notion of choice: kids get to make decisions on these play areas and then follow the conclusions to their natural end. They elect how to participate, assess, and manage their involvement As a result, each participant has a different experience. We will see more examples of children having immediate agency as we build on the notion of risk and mix it with the concepts of failing and succeeding. In order to fail or succeed, as we shall see in the next chapter, children have to sense that there has been a challenge to their status quo, that there is a possibility things could go wrong, but that they have the ability to take charge of the outcome.

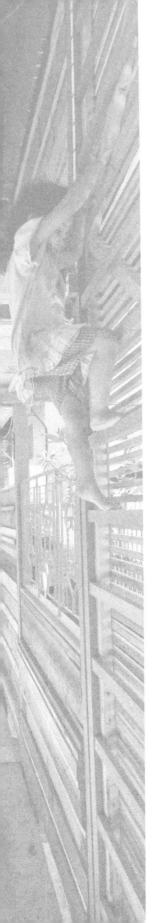

Failing and Succeeding

FAILURE AND MASTERY, both of which are discouraged in most American playgrounds, are the by-products of taking risks and pursuing activities for which there is no known outcome. In risk-free situations, children cannot demonstrate competence because they can do only what they already know they can achieve.[1] Chances for accomplishment and possible failure alter the dynamics of play and set the stage for activities that may be slightly more goal-focused, although the outcomes remain unclear. Mastery introduces success and reinforces a sense of personal achievement. Kids gain mastery when they succeed at a formidable task.[2]

Because mastery is such a pleasurable and self-sustaining event, children want to repeat exactly what they have just accomplished.[3] They push themselves a little harder with each success. Psychology professor Grolnick warns that parents should give their kids freedom to test their limits, otherwise they tend to give up too easily when they face a hard task.[4] Another psychologist maintains that when children fail and then bounce back to succeed, they "develop both the internal regulation and sense of agency that ultimately will allow them to make good choices about themselves, their health and their relationships."[5]

Sources

We are learning a great deal about failure and mastery from two different, albeit relatively new, fields: social cognitive development (SCD) and developmental cognitive neuroscience (DCN). Carol Dweck (professor of psychology at Stanford) is one of the pioneers of SCD. Dweck, who employs cognitive development research to understand social behavior,[6] has shown that children like to be challenged and don't enjoy tasks that are too easy. Dweck's research, although focused on student academic achievement, relates to personal growth, too. One of her main findings is that children need to believe that nothing (even IQ) is fixed or predetermined: if they have a "growth mind-set," they understand that they can push their own achievement through trial and error and hard work. She shows that this is as true for athletic accomplishment as for learning an academic subject.

Dweck's second, or corollary, finding is that students are helped if their parents, teachers, or coaches praise their effort rather than their prowess or accomplishment. That, too, leaves them room to improve.

Adele Diamond, who teaches at the University of British Columbia and has been a pioneer of DCN, writes that children gain self-confidence when they have the chance to do something hard and to succeed at it, even if it means making several failed attempts first.[7] They delight in overcoming difficult tasks. Once they succeed, they triumphantly take on even harder chores.[8] For both Dweck and Diamond, their findings suggest that rewarding actions are ongoing and never completed—which is the same way we would want to evaluate a playground.

Today's American playground rarely provides opportunities for children to fail and then push themselves to overcome their own limitations. American play spaces, having been eviscerated of risky challenges, are filled with activities that most kids can do without any struggle.

These same places are filled with parents who laud their children's success in climbing up a low four-step stairway or walking across an enclosed bridge that is raised only slightly above ground. It may not be possible to alter parents' behavior, although alerting them of what they are doing might be a good place to begin. It would also be useful to search for ways to confront children's abilities and to help them participate in difficult but not impossible actions. Let's hope that challenging playgrounds proliferate so that parents can say honestly to their offspring, "You really had to work to do that," instead of "You are the best climber in the world," when they did not have to exert themselves at all. It is heartening that many examples already exist that invite kids to try difficult but surmountable activities, and we can hope that their parents praise their efforts when they succeed.

Trees

Adults often remember (or claim to remember) childhood experiences of trees and tree climbing. Tree climbing offers an excellent opportunity for mastery because children have to make judgments about the sturdiness of the tree, about how high they want to travel, and where they eventually want to go. While an adventure at a suitable elevation is possible, most kids are pretty proud to have made the ascent. When children implore parents to create a tree hideaway for them, they seek special places to hang out; kids are certain that they are remote and secure in a place adults would not want to enter.

When tree houses occasionally pop up in today's public spaces, they

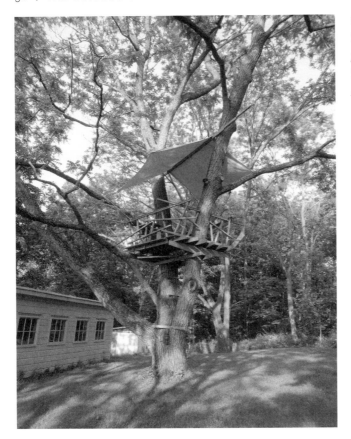

FIGURE 3.1
*Todd Rader + Amy Crews,
private tree house, upstate New
York. Courtesy of Todd Rader +
Amy Crews Architecture.*

usually have a gentle access route and high enclosures ring the top. Ramps or stairs make them accessible to all. It would be helpful if we could find a way to get all kids—disabled and fully mobile—to experience something more challenging, and again make the tree house a place of both accomplished arrival and sustained removal from parents or caregivers. More than thirty-five years ago environmental psychologists observed children pushing themselves in small increments to succeed in their outdoor environment. They point to a single tree as a source of continuing challenge, sustained even for years.[9]

It is possible to reinvigorate the design of the tree house so that it could be a useful part of public space. Todd Rader and Amy Crews, both of whom trained as architects and landscape architects (Todd Rader + Amy Crews Architecture Landscape Architecture), have updated several tree houses.[10] They look to a tree house they designed for a private client in Hudson, New York, as a sturdy model that could easily be adapted into a public venue. A larger deck, to hold many more than the six children who can fit into the private version, is not out of the question. The beauty of this simple abstraction is evident in the roof, meant to evoke a bird's nest, and in the limbs that follow the structure of a tree.

The best part of the Rader + Crews tree house is the climb along the side of the tree to get to the deck. If kids fail, they work on their skills until they get to the top. It's that simple. They have to plan and practice until they can get to the "house." Getting there is both the challenge and the fun. Because of the sloping ground, those who succeed are twelve to fifteen feet above the ground. The cost for these thrills and sense of achievement is modest, involving about $500 for materials for the private version. The designers feel that a similar structure for a park would probably be in the range of $8,000. A useful comparison is that a manufactured tree house, one with a small four-by-five-foot interior would have a price tag that exceeds $6,200 (before installation).

In a private kindergarten in the Tachikawa section of Tokyo, Japan, it is almost impossible to separate the playground and trees from the architecture of a school. With more than five hundred students, Fuji Montessori Kindergarten School (Tezuka Architects, 2007) is the largest kindergarten (ages two to six) in Japan.[11] Well-known graphic designer Kashiwa Sato (his clients have included Uniglo and Issey Miyake) brought architects Takaharu Tezuka and Yui Tezuka into the project.[12] Both members of this husband-and-wife team hold graduate degrees from the West: he went to the University of Pennsylvania and she to the Bartlett School of Architecture in London. They add their own take on Japanese values to modernism and Western practice, resulting in an aesthetic of fine craftsmanship, careful detailing, and wise use of seemingly modest natural materials. They talk about restoring "joy" and the full range of sensory experiences to children and incorporating those ideas into this school.

The Tezukas designed an oval, single-story, donut-shaped building that hugs an open central courtyard. The drawings of their own children, who spontaneously liked to draw circles, convinced the Tezukas that a circle or oval is a basic geometric form for which children have affection and understanding. It also was the ideal shape for replacing the old C-shaped school building that would be torn down. The new school has glass walls on all sides; the ones facing the courtyard are usually open. There are no interior divisions; lightweight furniture, which the children can move, provides the only demarcations of interior spaces.

The design of the building reflects the input of irrepressible principal Sekiichi Kato, whose ideas the Tezukas often had to tame. Kato, who tells

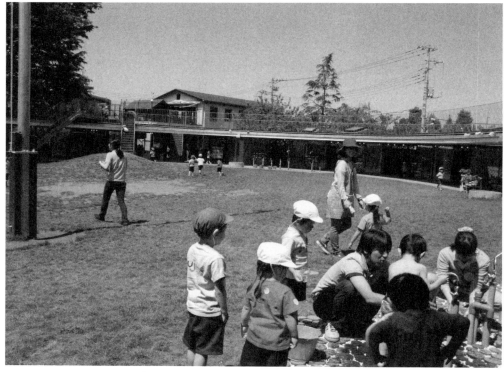

FIGURE 3.2 | *Tezuka Architects, Fuji Montessori School (2007), Tokyo, Japan. Running water, in the central play space, can be used for water play. In this photo, a teacher uses the water to wash a child who fell into the school's raised rice paddy. Author's photograph, 2013.*

parents that their child might break an arm or a leg at school but will never suffer a long-term injury such as head or neck fracture, wants kids to have chances for risk and the pleasure of success. The interior ceiling height is just over six feet in order to establish a "child scale." The short distance between the courtyard and flat roof above augments the connection between them, although the school principal would have liked it to have been even closer. The architects respected the school's request for a "roof house," a form that the Tezukas had explored in private homes but that has not been a popular notion in public space in Japan.

The courtyard and the roof, taken together, are effectively an enormous play site for climbing, sliding, and running. Teachers standing in the courtyard can actually monitor activity on the low roof and courtyard at the same time. From the courtyard, children can climb onto a sand mound and then ascend the stairs. Once on the roof, kids can run around or take the steep

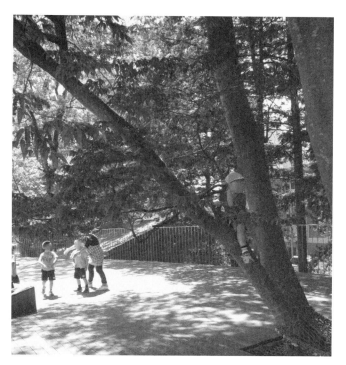

FIGURE 3.3
*Tezuka Architects, Fuji
Montessori School (2007), Tokyo,
Japan. Students can use the roof
to climb onto the three trees that
rise through it. They are free
to climb as high as they want.
Author's photograph, 2013.*

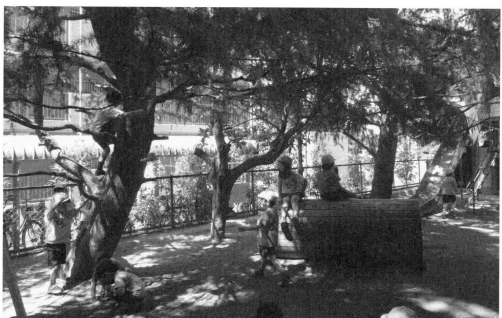

FIGURE 3.4 | *Tezuka Architects, Fuji Montessori School (2007), Tokyo, Japan.
This play section is on the exterior of the elliptical building, away from the entrance.
There are several trees, hollowed-out logs, high slides, climbing equipment, and
abundant sand on the ground. Author's photograph, 2013.*

slide back down to the courtyard. The roof is made of wood and is ideal for running or inventing games, and it has skylights so kids can peer into the classrooms (and the other way around). During quieter times, students can sit on the edge of the roof to watch a performance in the courtyard. It's large enough that the entire school could be out there at the same time. Kato would have preferred eliminating all hand rails along the roof. Forgoing them would have violated local building ordinances; so he countered with a suggestion to attach heavy netting to the building perimeter so that there would be a safe way to collect falling bodies. To satisfy the principal and to adhere to building codes, the architects chose the thinnest possible railing.

In another compromise with the principal's free spirit, the architects found a way to incorporate three existing trees into the roof scheme. These large zelkova trees serve as both infrastructure and play space. At the roof level, kids can climb down into a net that surrounds the trunk to have the sensation of grasping it, and then they can begin a climb up from the roof deck. Fisherman constructed the nets to ensure their strength; the architects feel that the netting captures Kato's first wish, to have children be safe while taking chances. Each tree is different, and kids can challenge themselves to be able to climb all three.

Vigorous activity also exists on the ground level at the back of the oval, the part farthest from the main gate. Since a low chain-link fence surrounds the school, there is leftover space for a "sand beach." Here there are more trees to climb, a hollowed out log to run through or hop on, and simple metal equipment for climbing and sliding. The expansive sand area blends into a section for water play. Continuing along this exterior part of the oval, there is a zone for plants and animals: two ponies live in a paddock, and rice and tea grow in some raised beds. Children casually come and go among all of these areas, including the space where they pet the ponies or touch the plants. They are free just to wander. If children should get dirty by falling into the rice paddy, they come into the courtyard where a teacher is ready to hose them down. Falling in the water is actually emblematic for this school, where kids are allowed to learn by making mistakes and then try again.

In 2011, Tezuka architects designed and completed an addition to the school that refines and expands some aspects of the first building. This round building houses English classes inside and a sheltered bus stop outside. The structure is a visual complement and excellent supplement to the oval shape of the main school. This smaller building, half-enclosed and half-open in accordance with the two needs it serves, is dominated by a single tree that occupies almost all of the space of the courtyard and extends above the roofline. Neither it nor the interstitial intermediate spaces that surround it are currently available for frolicking, but their presence reinforces the school's/principal's philosophy of exploration.

Nets

Tezuka Architects have designed another building, also in Japan, that protects a work of art where children test their mastery skills. Their collaboration, with fabric artist Toshiko Horiuchi MacAdam, is part of the permanent collection of the Hakone Open-Air Museum. Because this crocheted piece, Knitted Wonder Space II (2009), is on the grounds of a museum, there is an admission charge. The cost is reduced on Saturdays, when any adult can bring along up to five children or teens for free. It's not a no-cost neighborhood space, but membership possibilities exist for families to make affordable return visits.

MacAdam has a long association with this museum. Trained as a textile designer at Tama Fine Art University in Tokyo and at Cranbrook Academy in the United States, she originally thought of her fiber pieces as fine art.[13] In the 1970s, several children jumped into an installation of a fiber piece that filled an entire space that MacAdam had designed with a colleague. It was a career-altering event. MacAdam, who had been searching for a way to create a human connection within her art, saw that designing for kids would unite a piece made by hand with actual physical activity.

Intrigued by a new way to consider her own art, she set out with students to investigate how and where children play. Looking at Tokyo in the early 1970s, she saw that kids were cooped up in apartments, with few opportunities to be outside. It was a harsh reality that differed from the freedom she had growing up in Japan after World War II. Appropriately, she crocheted her first piece for children and gave it to a nursery school. In the early 1980s, she exhibited her fiber art at the Hakone Open-Air Museum; they subsequently commissioned her to design a piece for children for their permanent collection. This resulted in Knitted Wonder Space, an interactive sculpture made from braided nylon that she had hand dyed and crocheted. It was displayed inside a neutral gallery space where kids were not only allowed but also encouraged to play on it.

When the Hakone museum was celebrating its fortieth anniversary in 2009, it decided to replace Knitted Wonder Space with a new piece, again by MacAdam. MacAdam, who by now was working with her husband, Charles MacAdam, at their company, Interplay Design and Manufacturing in Canada, created an enlarged and updated version as Knitted Wonder

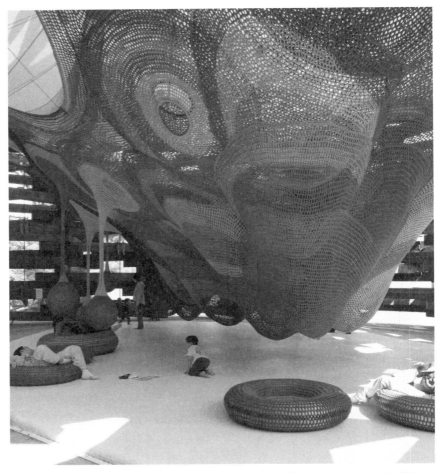

FIGURE 3.5 | *Toshiko Horiuchi MacAdam, Knitted Wonder Space II in Woods of Net pavilion designed by Tezuka Architects at Hakone Open Air Museum (2009), Hakone, Japan. The small openings ensure that the interior of the net is reserved for children. Author's photograph, 2013. (Plate 3)*

Space II. Both the first and second versions (and the Haugen/Zohar works in Trondheim) offer evidence that playscapes can be successful as pieces of art, with objects for playful activity, and in areas that demand children take a chance at surmounting obstacles. In the case of Knitted Wonder Space II, the attendance at the museum doubled as soon as it was installed. Families, especially those with young children, sometimes travel several hundred miles to spend a day on this knitted sculpture. Their excursions are testimony that this piece will keep children busy by challenging them to keep trying until they get higher and higher on the structure; if children were immediately successful, they and their parents would exit in a few minutes.

Knitted Wonder Space II is a hanging nylon piece that MacAdam has again dyed and crocheted herself. She asked engineer Norihide Imagawa to provide structural design. The resulting work resembles a suspended basket, one with protruding bulges at the bottom and a wide opening at the top. The MacAdams call it an "air pocket." The large colored circles of the overall design are eye popping. The suspended piece is augmented by crocheted hanging balls; crocheted round pillows rest below on the ground. The simple shapes, jolting colors, and beguiling knitted circles on the enormous net all entice children (who must be younger than twelve years old) to seek entry. The crochet weaves are open, so that kids who try to get inside can see (and hear) the other children who are already there. Their presence ensures that children first entering, who might have a tough time, will not give up.

Children (who have to take off their shoes, as this results in a better distribution of weight and tension) first climb up and into a small hole; it is a bit tricky, but its small size ensures that parents cannot enter behind. Holes close to the ground allow really small children to have a chance on this piece. Once through the initial entry, which hugs small bodies, kids have

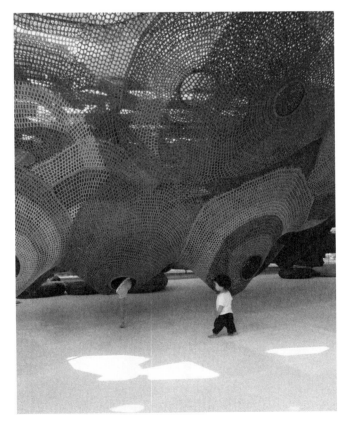

FIGURE 3.6
Toshiko Horiuchi MacAdam,
Knitted Wonder Space II
in Woods of Net pavilion
designed by Tezuka Architects
at Hakone Open Air Museum
(2009), Hakone, Japan.
Author's photograph, 2013.

to crawl along the side of the weaving until they arrive at a higher opening. They have to propel themselves through that in order to arrive at the broad interior of the crocheted piece. At that point, they have choices: they can climb farther and higher along the sides, or they can crawl or run across a large expanse. Children feel proud and successful when they reach the interior, and their delight continues when they see that they can manage different actions on the springy surface. Most important they realize that they are up high, where they can hang out and congregate with their peers and without direct parental control. They also have to figure out how to lower themselves down and out in order to reunite with parents or caregivers.

Tezuka Architects felt that MacAdam's piece should rest in an outdoor space, but they had to find ways to protect it from damage from rain and the sun. As a "protective construction," they came up with a freestanding, beehive-shaped pavilion ("Woods of Net") with wooden joints that evokes (seventeenth-century) Kiyomizu Temple in Kyoto. The 580 unique pieces of wood are arranged so that rainwater drains off. Wide spaces between the wood permit limited light to come in without removing a sense of secrecy. The pavilion has a sculptural quality that puts it at home on a site with many other pieces of outdoor sculpture, including works by Henry Moore and Joan Miro. If there were any way that this pavilion could have become a climbing structure, the architects would have gleefully adopted that concept.

Several of MacAdam's other net pieces are on exterior sites, including her early *Rainbow Hammock*. It is close to the Fog Forest in Showa Kinen Park. Her former student, landscape architect Fumiaki Takano (with whom she had collaborated on a piece for a national park in Okinawa), invited her to create something for the section of the park that he designed in the 1990s. She devised sixty-seven mechanically knotted nets, which she hand dyed. The nets start low to the ground, then overlap, but do not touch until at a height of ten or twelve feet. Since there is a slope to the rough ground, a child might be able to reach a high net quickly by first accessing it from a low spot. The colors change horizontally so that climbers can assess how far they have traveled from one side to another. Kids can bounce on the nets, but their major activity is climbing up and getting the thrill of mastering height. How to achieve this isn't always obvious; they have to plan each step of their journey. Instructions on a nearby sign indicate that this is for elementary school–age children and those even younger, but older kids and adults are always present. By dedicating this piece to young kids, the park encourages adults to use the surrounding ground plane as a picnic

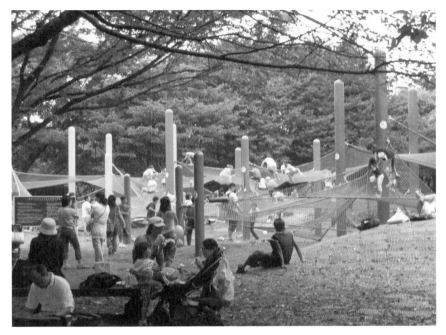

FIGURE 3.7 | *Toshiko Horiuchi MacAdam, Rainbow Hammock in Showa Kinen Park (1990), Tokyo, Japan. Fumiaki Takano, of Takano Landscape Planning, did the overall planning. The hammocks sit on dirt, where families enjoy picnics. Author's photograph, 2006.*

area where they can watch the kids from a distance. This family-oriented space rightfully becomes a space for families with young children, while teens flock to other parts of the park.

MacAdam sees all of her pieces as organic; every six to eight years there are major repairs. It fits well with the Japanese tradition of continually repairing the interior shoji screens in a home; it also meshes with the Shinto belief in the ongoing life and death of holy objects, including the sacred shrine at Ise, which is replaced every twenty years.

MacAdam's pieces are specific to each client. An entirely different net, one that is industrial and not necessarily visually tied to its site, challenges kids and adults in Saratoga Springs, Utah. This particular piece—called Neptun xxl by its manufacturer, Berliner-Seilfabrik—could seem anxiety producing, but it has shown that people of all ages respond to a chance to conquer what might at first appear to be difficult.[14] It also indicates that a town can look to a play area to give it a distinctive identity.

In this case, Saratoga Springs was, until 1997, an area of unincorporated suburbs outside of Salt Lake City. Like its namesake in upstate New York, the town bills itself as a resort area and features natural hot springs and spas. Having grown from one thousand to more than seventeen thousand people between 2000 and 2012, this small city expects to continue rapid growth. The municipal leaders sought an iconic centerpiece. After creating a ten-acre park that includes a harbor and boat launch, they sought a memorable marker. They were thinking of perhaps something reminiscent of an old Ferris wheel or a carousel, which could bring together citizens of all ages. They settled on Neptun XXL, because of its considerable height (thirty feet) and distinctive pyramidal shape. It is not a unique piece but is the first to arrive in the Western Hemisphere. And while its cost may seem high (over $180,000 before installation), it accommodates many people for hours

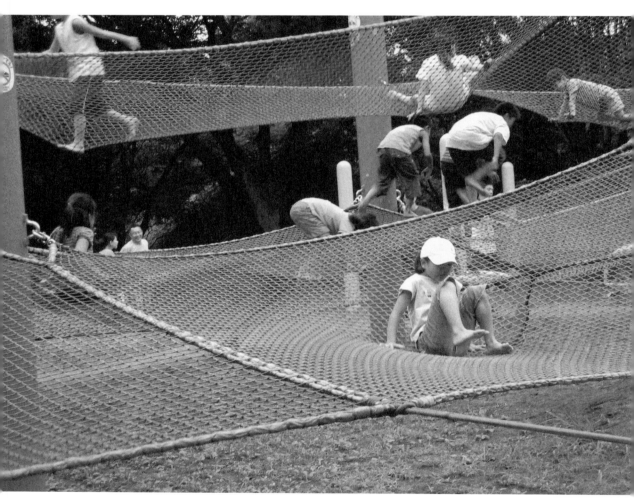

FIGURE 3.8 | *Toshiko Horiuchi MacAdam, Rainbow Hammock in Showa Kinen Park (1990), Tokyo, Japan. Author's photograph, 2006.*

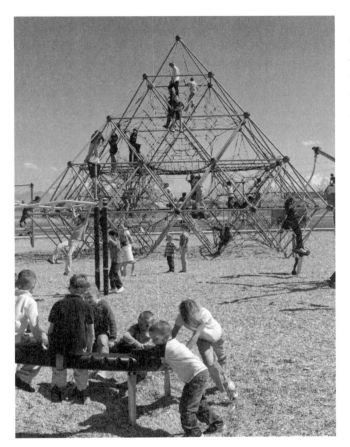

FIGURE 3.9

Gregory H. Graves, Landscape Architect and J-U-B-Engineers (2011). Neptun XXL pyramid climber (Berliner Seilfabrik), in Neptune Park, Saratoga Springs, UT. Photography by Alyse.

each day. Smaller versions of similar rope climbers—now found on many American playgrounds—seem to have the ability to pull in many children simultaneously and to give them a chance to first fail and then succeed.

Despite all appearances, the Neptun net is actually quite safe. The city does not maintain an age restriction, nor is the installation fenced. City managers say that parents can put any child on the net as soon as the parents are comfortable doing so. Interior netting means that all falls are cushioned and no single fall can be more than six feet. If a small child falls from a low height, he has to look around and figure out a better way to do it the next time. For kids, the Neptun xxL provides a chance to challenge themselves to go higher and higher. Older folks, especially those who have watched small kids conquer the contraption, come at night to have a try getting to the top. Lighting and the nearby lake make this an attractive public space in which adults can gather. City officials, so pleased with the buzzing activity and with a sense that the former subdivision is now identified by a demanding play structure, have appropriated the equipment name for the entire area, which is now Neptune Park.

Domes

Adriaan Geuze, a founder of the landscape and urban design firm West 8 in Rotterdam, spoke at a Museum of Modern Art symposium in 2012. The subject was "The Child in the City of Play."[15] Geuze showed an image of the Borneo Sporenburg section of Amsterdam, where West 8 did the master plan. He focused on a very high bridge he specified for the project. It is over a part of the canal system where only low boats travel. He quickly added that he wanted the bridge to be unnecessarily high so that local children could use it to jump into the water and create their own fun. It was a fascinating admission that demonstrates how planning for kids may be both easier and more subtle than expected. It is possible, too, that children are aware of play possibilities and paths to mastery that their parents do not grasp.

Jørgen Moe, a ceramicist who also teaches at Queen Maud University in Trondheim, shows how kids can accept challenges that adults might not see immediately. He creates domes and takes advantage of weather conditions in the part of the playground he designed at Nedre Flatåsen Barnehage. This is a new kindergarten, completed in 2010, in a residential section of Trondheim. Moe's contribution to the playground is art, like so many other pieces in kindergartens in Trondheim, and was supported by the city's Percent for Art program. Inspired by the broken ceramics wedged into concrete at Antonio Gaudi's Park Guell in Barcelona, Moe created a series of low domes covered with colorful tiles.

The domes are sturdy enough for children to climb onto, and maybe even to slip off. In the warm months, one dome has a small fountain that spouts water. Stone paths connect the domes, giving kids a chance to see how the water trickles over the stones; they can crawl or ride bikes on the uneven surfaces. They can devise their own running or racing games. In the wintery months, which begin in October, the domes are often half hidden by snow. Teachers can activate a computer chip that controls light emitting from each sphere. The lights remind the children that the domes are still available for climbing and sitting; they can also be used as the centerpiece for digging into the snow or piling snow into even higher mounds. Accordingly, the children get very excited when the lights go on and they realize that they can, again, test themselves on these mounds.

Taking the "dome" theme to a different material and a larger scale, landscape architects Michael van Valkenburgh Associates (MVVA) used a

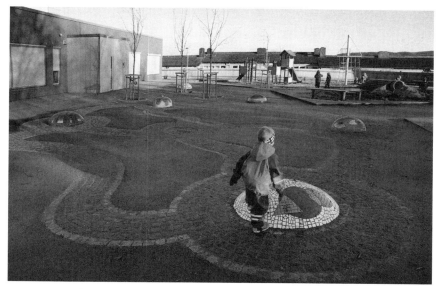

FIGURE 3.10 | *Jørgen Moe, ceramic domes and pebble paths for Nedre Flatåsen Barnehage (2012), Trondheim, Norway. Courtesy of Jørgen Moe. Photograph by Grethe B. Fredriksen.*

high-stainless version in Union Square Park in New York City. MVVA chose a great deal of equipment, including some directly off the shelf, for the refurbishment of this playground. The outstanding piece of the playground is a large, stainless-steel dome made by the Goric Marketing Group USA. Located in the corner farthest from the entrance and from the section for small children, the dome appears to be the most successful piece of equipment there. Preteens and teens try to get to the top with one jump, or they jump on and then work their way to the top. They egg each other on to see if they can get to the top in a single sprint. Those on top glow in their accomplishment, and urge their friends to join them; they even encourage younger children to have a try. They further test their abilities by inventing new ways to master the slope. Some will try to "walk" down the steep incline without falling; others see if they can slide down on their stomach. A five-year-old from New Hampshire, visiting her grandparents who live nearby, insisted on coming to the dome every day: she tried to climb it each time and was not satisfied until she finally got to the top. In all of these instances, kids of varying ages set their own goals and then struggled to achieve them.

In spite of the large dome's success, the same designer's experience with smaller versions of the domes led to a less happy outcome. MVVA called for three small domes, each two feet high, in their plan for Brooklyn Bridge Park

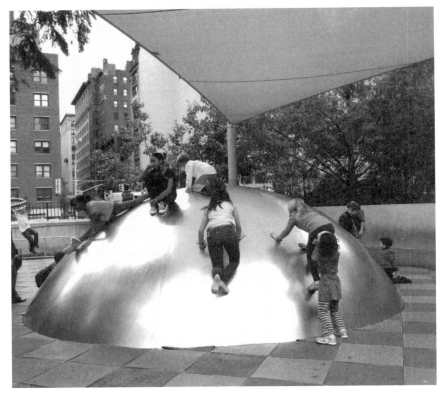

FIGURE 3.11 | *Michael van Valkenburgh Associates used this large Goric stainless steel dome "mountain" for the Union Square Playground (2011), New York City. The awning helps to reduce buildup of heat on the metal. Author's photograph, 2012.*

(Pier 6 section). The low domes are the perfect size for small fry and offered them a different climbing experience than what is usually available in American playgrounds. The Brooklyn domes arrived in March 2010 for the small kiddie section in this eighty-five-acre, $350 million park developed by the state. Within a few months, as the weather got warmer, the domes heated up. Accusations soon followed that kids were burning their hands. Many local parents became indignant. By mid-June, the Empire State Development agency had fenced off the domes and covered them with a tarp; by the end of the month, the agency had replaced them with low, standard-issue equipment.[16]

In the name of safety and responding to angry parents, the state agency had lost a chance to give kids a way to learn from their experiences. Admittedly, the landscape architect should have thought about providing some shade covering; it will be some time before nearby trees mature. Even so, removing the domes altogether seems extreme. Perhaps the park's administrators could have responded to the parents by saying, "We know you are afraid your child will get scorched, but there is a way to look at these domes as teaching aids." Kids approach them; if they are hot, children should know to take their hands off. A playground is a real place, and kids should not expect every single piece to be immune to local conditions.

Unexpected Materials

If parents can fault stainless equipment for being unsafe in warm weather, the future looks troubling for designers. One solution for them might be, for the sake of expediency and lowering costs, to look to materials that were never intended for play. These often present mastery challenges in unexpected ways.

Architect Katie Winter has built a practice that transforms ordinary building supplies into play opportunities for students at cash-strapped schools in New York City. Immaculate Conception School in the Bronx (pre-K to eighth grade) commissioned Winter to bring some cohesion to a large, somewhat unruly site. She came up with an appealing strategy. She transformed an abandoned swimming pool — too expensive to remove — into a filled-in space that rises to create a small hill. She also used ground pavers so that kids can jump from one to the other. She created a high garden folly using only chain link fence and poles.

Since all the students use all of the space (and almost half of the more than seven hundred students can be on the playground at one time), Winter had to devise solutions that were appropriate for diverse ages. She turned again to poles, the kind that hold up chain link fences, and used them to transform another part of the play area. She had the poles powder-coated red and blue and she placed them on a grid. From face on, they appear as a single layer; from the center of the space it appears to be a more spacious precinct than it really is. The children have transformed this simple arrangement into a play area where they come to invent new games and get better at the ones they have already developed. They find ways to roll balls among the poles; they swing from them; and most daringly, they swing and release, so that they get a sense of "flying." Flying is risky and exhilarating, but it is also something they have to practice to get right. Not surprisingly, students from all age groups flock to this play section.

For a schoolyard that also functions as a public park but was an asphalt lot in Rotterdam, architects Monica Adams and Juliette Bekkering (Bekkering Adams Architecten) used a bold piece of "equipment" to serve the needs of the diverse residents, young and old, who live nearby.[17] The city site sat

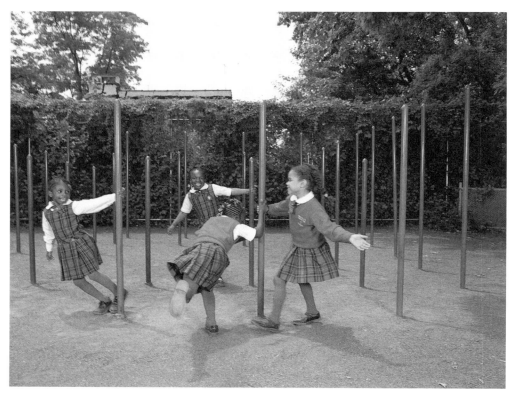

FIGURE 3.12 | *Katie Winter Architecture with Bothwell Site Design, Immaculate Conception School (2010), New York City. Photograph by and courtesy of Carl Posey Photo.*

on a pier, Mullerpier, next to a public school dedicated to technology and the theater arts. After setting aside an enclosed sports zone for active athletics, including basketball, the architects focused on distinct seating arrangements for both adults and kids in different areas of the schoolyard.

Their most intriguing design decision also involved seating, but in an unanticipated way. In the area for the younger children, the architects specified a commercially available piece of "landscape furniture"—and they flipped it upside down. Barcelona architects EMBT (Enric Miralles—Benedetta Tagliabue) had designed the piece and dubbed it "Lungo Mare." It has been available to the public (Escofet is the manufacturer) since 2000. Reflecting the rise and fall of waves, the piece comes in three modular sections, each weighing more than three thousand pounds. With its weight and smooth, polished surface, made from reinforced cast stone, Lungo Mare is both indestructible and unmovable. Bekkering Adams saw the potential of using just a single module, available at a relatively low cost of €8,000 ($10,400), as a piece of playground equipment.

The imagery of waves is not inappropriate for a space that is on an old pier. By reversing the seat's position, Bekkering Adams accentuated the deep bowl in the center and created a high, cantilevered arm. Small children need to figure out how to climb up onto the arm, and then how to jump off once they're on. They often need several tries to accomplish this. Will they jump from a high point, or go back to the section closest to the ground? No matter what they decide, kids have to master horizontal and vertical dimensions. The abstract design encourages them to come up with fantastic scenarios; they can indulge in a variety of sociodramatic events suggesting a spaceship or pirate boat. While the playground does include a more traditional piece of climbing equipment, the kids gravitate to the upside-down seating piece.

The school is diligent about providing balls and jump ropes, simple implements that let the children create their own play systems. Here the surface, one part of which remains asphalt alongside a larger flat rubber section, is integrated well together. Neither material is very satisfactory separately, but together they accommodate this small schoolyard and

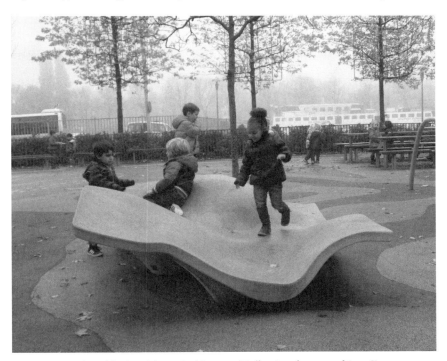

FIGURE 3.13 | *Bekkering Adams Architecten, Mullerpier playground (2008), Rotterdam, Netherlands. This piece of "equipment" is the Lungo Mare bench (Escofet, 2000) that architects Enric Miralles and Benedetta Tagliabue (EMBT) designed. Author's photograph, 2012.*

encourage interactive activities among students. Asphalt surfacing may still have a place in schoolyards for traditional ball games, jump rope, and for chalk drawings. On some American playgrounds, it is still necessary as a place where kids line up before entering the building and as the site where hopscotch occurs: in the twenty-first century, hopscotch in the United States — perhaps because it has become somewhat rare — has lost its gender bias and both young boys and girls seem to like it.

Accessibility

In the United States, we tend to think of "accessibility" as ways in which to conform to the Americans with Disabilities Act (ADA). Passed in 1990 and later amended, ADA has precise requirements for playgrounds so that disabled children, especially those in wheelchairs, can be accommodated. While important, ADA is not perfect. It does not always provide sufficiently for nonwheelchair disabilities, such as lack of hearing or sight. Those impairments equal the number of wheelchair confinements in children and teens. Issues of accessibility for very small children or the poor are also out of its purview. Some designers are now, fortunately, thinking about how to address accessibility for those with varied physical disabilities, those who are very young, and even those who live in poor urban enclaves. The designers strive to integrate diverse populations so that all public space is shared.

Landscape architect Helle Nebelong, a long-time advocate for challenging play spaces, found many opportunities for stimulating the actions of kids — including those with disabilities — when she redesigned a playground in her native Copenhagen.[18] Her playground, once the site of the city dump and subsequently an adventure playground, is in Valby Park, one of the largest public spaces in the country. The city, which restored the park as part of its preparations for its role as the European Culture Capital of 1996, built seventeen gardens on the site. The playground is one of them.

Nebelong's site required the soil remediation of more than three feet of then-current surface. It had to be removed before she could begin her project. The removed dirt, which had to stay in the park, was perfect for creating a series of hillocks that could then be covered with clean earth. These artificial hills created an opportunity to produce a landscape that could offer variation without purchasing equipment. Some areas emphasize rocks, while others highlight sand, the foliage of dense brush, or irregular shapes of driftwood. There are willow huts and a meadow.

Two elements of particular note address mastery: the use of dead trees

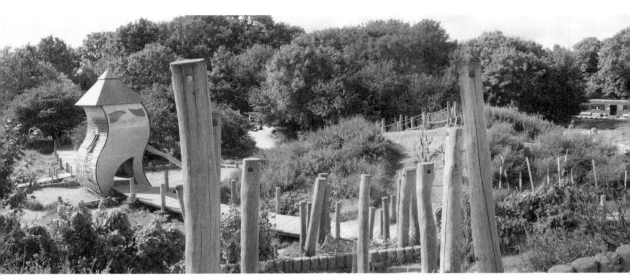

FIGURE 3.14 | *Helle Nebelong, Valby Park (2001), Copenhagen. Courtesy of Helle Nebelong Landscape Architect. Photograph by Helle Nebelong.*

and the full accessibility of the park. Nebelong organized the space within a foot-and-a-half-high circular boardwalk, created from elm trees that had died on this site. The boardwalk is just high enough for children to jump off or hide under. For small kids, it poses a chance to overcome a scary height. Elsewhere in the park, Nebelong has taken advantage of dead trees by using them horizontally as climbing apparatuses. No two are alike, and several offer kids a chance to climb high and dangle from extended branches. For children who come often, the trees must be a place to return to and keep trying to reach particular heights.

The park is accessible for the handicapped, yet there are no paved or smooth paths. Nebelong expects those who are blind or in wheelchairs to make their way up the dirt or pebble paths, especially the snail-shaped one that goes to the top of a hill. She believes that all people should be challenged, including those with disabilities. She often cites the legacy of adventure playgrounds as an important aspect of how she designs. Believing that adventure playgrounds permitted kids to "train themselves in dealing with and triumphing over unpredictability," she now tries "to accomplish the same thing using water, sand, soil, stones, plants, terracing, and hidden spaces among natural growing materials."[19]

Very young children are another group that does not often have access to interesting public play sites. They are usually relegated to simplistic equipment that they quickly outgrow. Carve, the designers in Amsterdam who

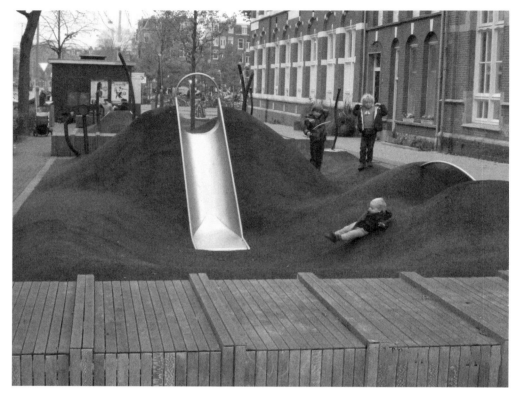

FIGURE 3.15 | *Carve, play street on Potgieterstraat (2010), Amsterdam, Netherlands. Author's photograph, 2012.*

created the Vondel Park towers, have come up with a winning streetscape that addresses mastery without hazard; in the process, it helps to create new communities, including ones for the youngest and oldest possible users.[20] This particular streetscape on Potgieterstraat is also an elegant version of traffic calming, a goal at the heart of many new urban design plans.[21]

The project, which began in 2007, was completed in 2010. The local municipality asked three firms to pitch ideas for taming a small street that had active traffic. It soon became clear that the local stakeholders—neighbors of varying ages, concerned parents, and a school—had varying and sometimes conflicting dreams for the street. Their wish lists included a playground for the school (which ultimately moved); areas for sports, including football, skating, water play, and basketball; green space; retention of ten to twelve existing parking spaces; and bicycle parking. The budget, €200,000 ($260,000), seemed small for a fifteen-hundred-square-meter space.

Carve had to sift through all of these often conflicting wishes. After conducting extensive interviews, Carve decided to turn the street into a

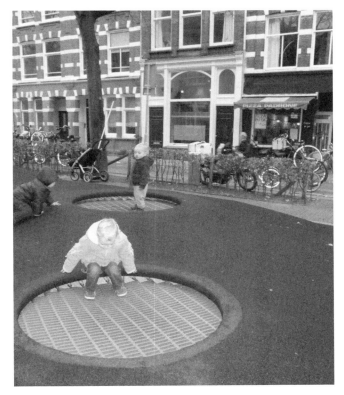

FIGURE 3.16

Carve, play street on
Potgieterstraat (2010),
Amsterdam, Netherlands.
Author's photograph, 2012.

dedicated play space for both ends of the age spectrum. Carve focused on a play space for very young kids along with seating that would be enticing for older folks. Their goal was to find ways to incorporate undirected play into kids' lives while also giving them opportunities to try to master age-appropriate amenities. The final hurdle was persuading (per municipal ordinance) 70 percent of some fifteen hundred nearby households to support the plan. Carve accomplished that by pointing out to residents how their scheme connected to the local community's appreciation of young and old individuals.

The result (a far cry from using a few road cones to mark off a "play street") is best for very small children: six to eighteen months old. It corrects a common problem. Small children — pretoddlers — cannot do much on a playground, even one that has been streamlined for kids six months to two years old. These young visitors are not ready for sand and might not be completely steady on their feet. They need to test their skills, but most of these playgrounds have stairs they might not be able to handle, or decks that are a bit too high. At the same time, infants need to fall in order to learn how to be upright.[22] Recent research on locomotion shows that infants and

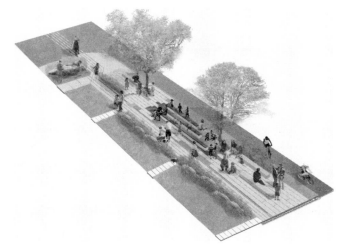

FIGURE 3.17
Marpillero Pollak Architects,
streetscape from competition
entry, Movement on Main:
A Design Competition for the
Healthy Main Street, (2013),
Syracuse, New York. Courtesy
of Marpillero Pollak Architects.

toddlers are "always learning to learn to move."[23] In very young children, repetition is a type of mastery.[24]

This play street is lively and welcoming. The houses on each side of Potgieterstraat are enclosing elements for the long, narrow site. Bikes on a bike path, parallel to the houses, are now the only traffic. The "play street" is broken into two sections, thereby allowing twice the number of benches on each of the short ends. Instead of fences, the play space uses people as barriers if a child should wander off. Older folks in the neighborhood sit and chat with friends at the end of the day. Caregivers also sit while their kids play; they are close enough if needed but far enough to let the children feel independent.

Low hills break the flat surface on both ends of the play street. Throughout, the surface is made of EPDM granules, a synthetic rubber made of recycled materials. Any toddler (or even an infant who crawls) should be able to get on and off these gentle mounds. The undulating surfaces feature hills of differing heights and widths so that little folks can repeat the experience without replicating the exact same route. Some of the hills are even large enough to hide behind. Additional treats — such as embedded small trampolines and tunnels and an embanked low slide — can be accessed by children of various ages. Tiny tots can take off on their own for small distances. For older kids, up to about eight or ten years old, the surface is very good for making chalk drawings or marking off games they invent. They also like to hang out on the low hills, jump on the trampolines, or talk to each other through the sound pipes.

A few American cities are considering how to reunite isolated, especially poorer, areas with central parts of a downtown. In Syracuse, New York, Marpillero Pollak Architects won honorable mention for their entry in the Movement on Main: A Design Competition for the Healthy Main competition. Although they did not secure the top designation, Marpillero Pollak still created a positive stir because of their attempt to uncover the local natural and economic histories of the area—including salt marshes and bicycle manufacturing. They also envisioned an urban trail along Wyoming Street, the main street of a former industrial zone ("Near Westside") that has long been separated from the downtown by an expressway and a polluted canal. They designed a meandering linear park that would have had grassy hills, rocks, plants, and water.

Marpillero Pollak saw an opportunity to create urban trails that would lead from Wyoming Street to secure ways to cross the trafficked or polluted areas. The trail was not identical to Wyoming Street; it was a new interventional path that wove in and out of it. There would be natural plantings on both sides of the street. The designers wanted to have lots of areas for stopping, resting, and chatting with neighbors. For young and old, they hoped to create "play pods." These would have had seating as well as free-form objects (including irregular rocks) that children could test themselves on by climbing or, where they could take a chance, by jumping. There could have been small, semisecluded nooks for play, too. The goal was to create different ways that residents could be energetic within the trail and effectively activate Wyoming Street while also having entry to other parts of the city.

Marpillero Pollak's entry, like the other projects in this section, shows the dual aspects of failing and succeeding: a site can be engaging and calm, but there has to be room for disquiet, the unknown. Children should never look at playgrounds and know the precise route or accomplishment they will achieve; there should always be a sense of unclear outcome, along with the ability to triumph over failed attempts. These projects, as well as those that entail some form of risk, are straightforward, and as we have seen, often quite affordable and possibly multigenerational. Our quest becomes more abstract—and sometimes harder to pin down—when we try to apply executive function to the public realm.

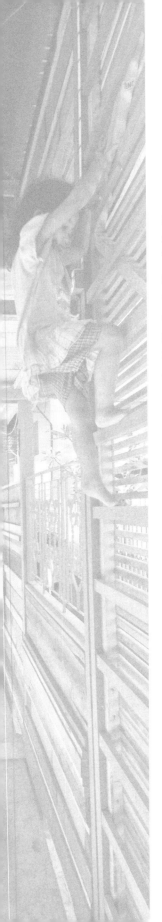

Executive Function

MANY CONTEMPORARY SCIENTIFIC investigations of children's neurocognitive development focus on something called "executive function" (EF). Tied to the neural circuitry of the brain's prefrontal cortex, EF is not a single action, nor does it have a sole identifying characteristic.[1] It is a fluid concept (not unlike play) with several evolving definitions. Despite some differences, most researchers agree that it involves self-control, delayed gratification, and the ability to ignore distractions, stay on task, and forgo impulsive behavior.[2] They also believe it encompasses doing several things at once, making mental connections, and being intellectually flexible. The EF domain includes sequencing, planning, and problem-solving. One of the most distinguished investigators of the concept, Adele Diamond, has tried to streamline the discussion of EF by creating a two-pronged hierarchical definition. She distinguishes between the main core executive functions—inhibitory control, cognitive flexibility, and working memory—and their complex achievements—problem solving, reasoning, and planning.[3]

EF in Action

Researchers claim that EF is essential for academic success and emotional health, as well as for the best long-term outcomes of career and marriage.[4] Diamond and her colleagues show that the EF of young children outranks reading and math as key components to academic success.[5] Other researchers have linked EF to "social-emotional competence."[6] There is some evidence that eight-year-olds who perform well on EF testing, when they become teens, are better able to problem-solve when on a team, and, as individuals, are better able to resolve conflicts with their parents.[7]

Other psychologists, while not directly addressing EF, write about self-control. Martin E. P. Seligman and Angela Duckworth have written about how self-discipline can shape outcomes; self-discipline was more important than IQ in predicting academic performance.[8] Think, too, about Walter Mischel and his famous marshmallow experiments in the late 1960s and early 1970s. Mischel asked four-year-olds to look at two marshmallows. They could eat one immediately, or, those who waited for a researcher

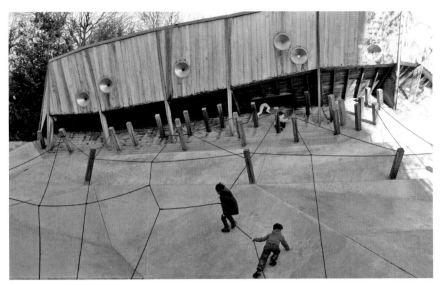

PLATE 1 | *BASE Landscape Architects, playground in Belleville Park, Paris, 2008. This is the playground at its lowest point. Children use ropes to hoist themselves up to the enclosed area under the wood facing. Photograph by Robert S. Solomon, 2012.*

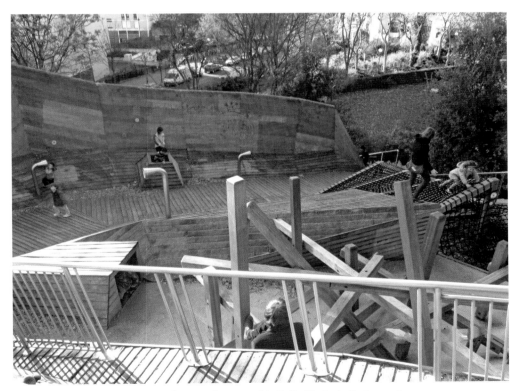

PLATE 2 | *BASE Landscape Architects, playground in Belleville Park, Paris, 2008. This is the second higher level, where children reach the wooden terrace of the playground. Photograph by Robert S. Solomon, 2012.*

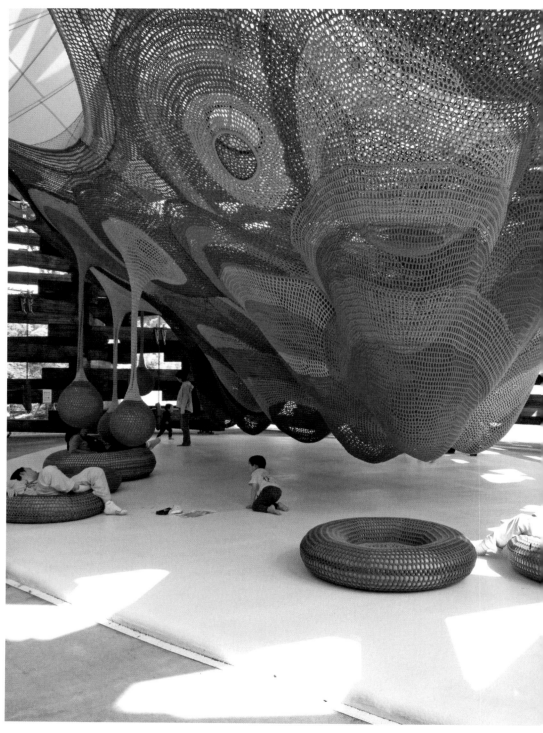

PLATE 3 | *Toshiko Horiuchi MacAdam, Knitted Wonder Space II in Woods of Net pavilion designed by Tezuka Architects at Hakone Open Air Museum (2009), Hakone, Japan. The small openings ensure that the interior of the net is reserved for children. Author's photograph, 2013.*

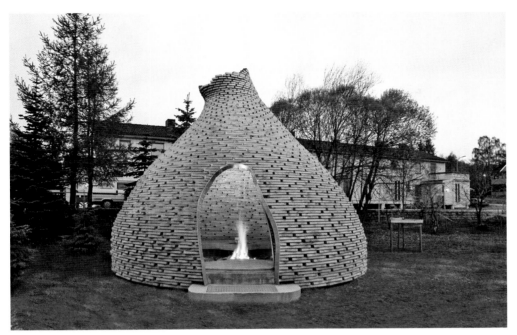

PLATE 4 | *Haugen/Zohar Arkitekter, exterior of fire pit at Skjaermveien Barnehage (2009), Trondheim, Norway.* The Architectural Review *chose this for an award in its 2009 AR+D Emerging Architecture program. Courtesy of Haugen/Zohar Arkitekter.*

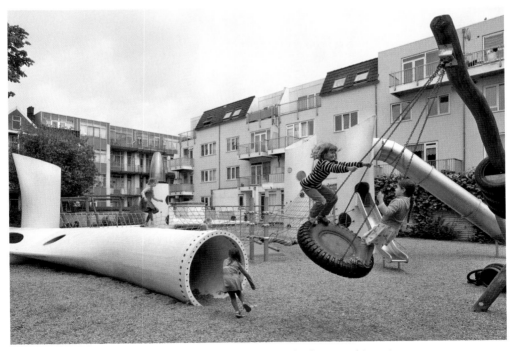

PLATE 5 | *2012Architecten (now Superuse Studios), Wikado playground (2009), Rotterdam, Netherlands. Photograph by and courtesy of Denis Guzzo.*

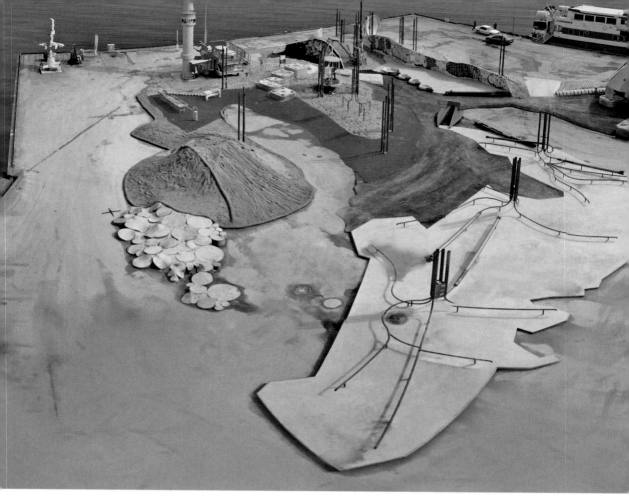

PLATE 6 | *Helen & Hard, Geopark (2008), Stavanger, Norway.*
Courtesy of Helen & Hard. Photograph by Emile Ashley.

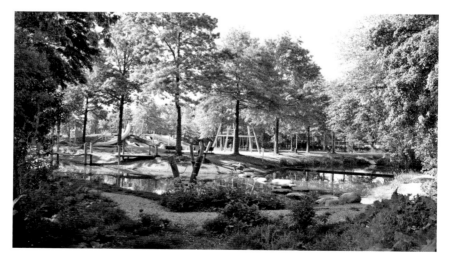

PLATE 7 | *Carve, Meer Park (2010), Amsterdam. There are areas for play*
on both banks of the stream. Courtesy of Carve.nl.

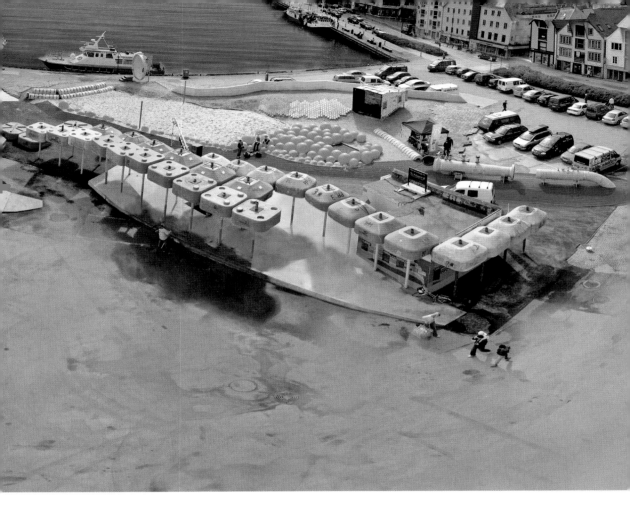

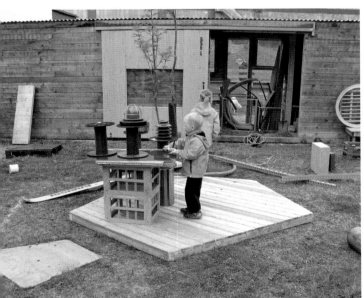

PLATE 8

Brendeland & Kristoffersen, outdoor space at Svartlamon Kindergarten (2007), Trondheim, Norway. The view is from the recycling center (next door) with a view toward the sheep that stay at the school and the playground hill, beyond. Courtesy of Pål Bøyesen and ReMida, Trondheim.

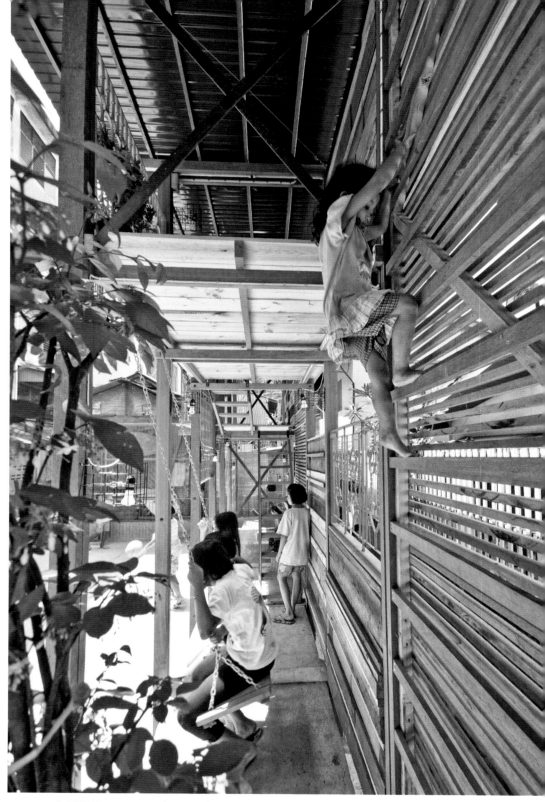

PLATE 9 | *TYIN Tegnestue Architects, Klong Toey Community Lantern (2011),*
Bangkok, Thailand. Photo by Pasi Aalto. Courtesy of TYIN Tegnestue Architects.

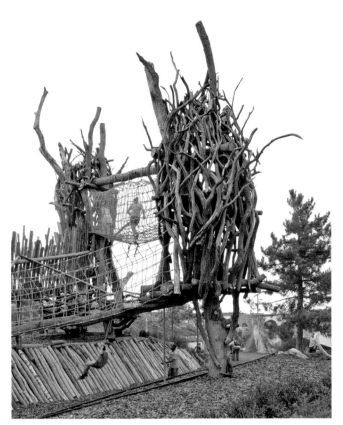

PLATE 10

erect architecture (playstructure) and LUC (design landscaping) (2013), Queen Elizabeth Olympic Park north playground, London. This project won the competition that the London Legacy Development Corporation sponsored for one of the sites left following the 2012 Olympic Games. Photograph by David Grandorge. Courtesy of erect architecture.

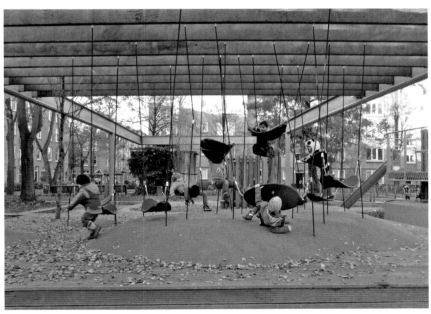

PLATE 11 | *Concrete Architects, Dijk & Co. landscape architects, and Carve. Van Beuningenplein (2011), Amsterdam, Netherlands. Carve designed this ingenious climbing device by reconfiguring sling swings. Author's photograph, 2012.*

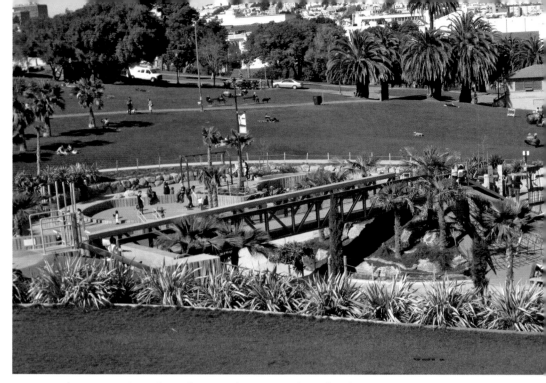

PLATE 12 | *Steven Koch, Koch Landscape Architecture. Helen Diller Playground at Dolores Park (2012), San Francisco, CA. The playground fits into the deep bowl of the park and is hardly visible to cars passing by on the street. Author's photograph, 2013.*

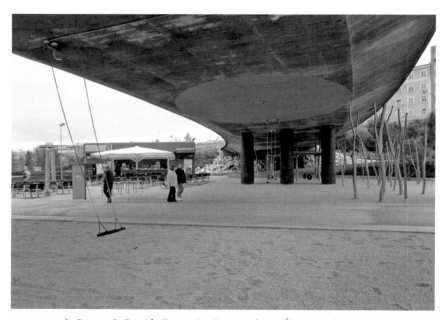

PLATE 13 | *Burgos & Garrido/Porras La Casta/Rubio & Álvarez-Sala/West 8; Team Director: Ginés Garrido, Madrid Rio (2011), Madrid, Spain. The swings, suspended from a red bullseye under the bridge, evoke Aldo van Eyck's use of "leftover" spaces to support activities for children. This view also shows how other play areas, a cafe, and a walking, jogging trail are interwoven seamlessly. Photograph by Robert S. Solomon, 2013.*

to "run an errand" could have two upon his return. Mischel followed up with the children as teens in the 1980s, and later as adults. Those who restrained themselves were the ones to succeed educationally, economically, and socially.[9] These psychologists confirm theories that go back to the early twentieth century, when Lev Vygotsky had proposed that motivation and cognition were intertwined in self-regulation.[10]

New imaging technologies are giving us more information about how and where EF takes place. We know, for instance, that the prefrontal cortex is the perfect location on which to effect change. Reporter Paul Tough has summarized why that is so: "The prefrontal cortex is more responsive to intervention than other parts of the brain, and it stays flexible well into adolescence and early adulthood."[11] We also now know a bit about the mechanics: delayed gratification is the result of developing and refining the dorsolateral prefrontal cortex so that it can electrically be strategic in how it activates the ventromedial prefrontal cortex.[12] A somewhat more simplified version recognizes the role of the prefrontal cortex, which is believed to direct goals, and the anterior cingulate cortex, which "is activated by tasks that require cognitive control."[13]

The playground may seem like the wrong place to encourage self-control or delayed gratification. Arguing for inhibitory control might, after all, look like an endorsement of the way kids wait for a chance to climb on a post and deck system. But such default thinking denies the complexity of EF. The metal domes that caused such an uproar at Brooklyn Bridge Park are a fine example of how delayed gratification might work in open space. If the domes were still present, kids would have to identify the problem if the domes were too hot and come up with an alternative activity until the domes cooled.

We tend to be nostalgic about children who were able to roam their neighborhoods and make their own fun as groups of kids in the 1950s and 1960s. Even if we may have an inflated appreciation for those times, we can recognize how children had to exercise EF skills. When those kids banded together to build a fort or a playhouse, they were being focused and flexible. They concentrated on what they were doing, and made up their own script; they decided informally what they would construct and, together, they designated who would manage each of the jobs necessary to complete the final product. Inhibitory control and cognitive flexibility would have been evident in the give and take of working together, learning to compromise, staying on task. In contrast, the post and deck system of today does not harbor unintentional or unknown outcomes, and it does not force kids to work together. Awareness of how EF can exist on a playground shows that it would not be impossible or onerous to bring back some opportunities to exercise it.

Fire and Water: Norway and Australia

In Norway and Australia, two distinctly different cultures, local demands have shaped how designers create areas where children have to exercise self-control and careful planning.

A day care and preschool (Skjaermveien Barnehage) in Trondheim, Norway, wanted to add to their playground.[14] They already had a hill (ubiquitous on Norwegian playgrounds) for climbing, sliding, and skiing; they had swings; and they had the deep, overhanging roof found on most kindergarten buildings: the place where infants nap in their carriages, semiprotected from the harshest temperatures.

The facility lacked an area where kids could play quietly in a confined space, listen to a story, sit around a campfire, and toast their sandwiches for lunch. The Oslo firm Haugen/Zohar (the same firm that designed the Cave, also in Trondheim) came up with a Fire Hut design that is sophisticated, resourceful, and a smart homage to the turf huts that are scattered throughout the Norwegian landscape. It allows children to develop important skills of self-control. The project, completed in 2009,[15] is another work that the local Percent for Art program funded. Once again, the price, at 350,000 Norwegian krone (approximately $60,000), was a good investment. The kids get to inhabit a unique work of art and, given the vigorous use of outdoor space in Norway, they use the Fire Hut daily.[16]

The architects had the benefit of inexpensive or redundant materials nearby. Taking advantage of local wood construction, they secured leftover pieces from a nearby building site. They specified eighty courses of pine planks, with oak spacers that diminish in length as they go higher.[17] The conical hut (approximately fifteen feet in diameter) becomes smaller and slightly irregular as it gets higher and reaches its eventual height of four meters (thirteen feet). The exterior blends in with the winter snow; light filters through the open spaces between planks into the interior. At the heart of the hut is a fire pit that sits beneath the off-center opening at the top. The aperture augments the wall openings to remind children that nature is just outside. A concrete base hugs and stabilizes the wood walls; it surrounds the fire and provides a free-form ledge where kids can sit and chatter around the fire. The entire arrangement is not unlike what Americans think of as a campfire setting.

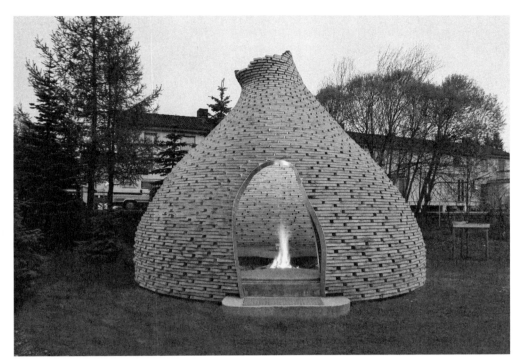

FIGURE 4.1 | *Haugen/Zohar Arkitekter, exterior of fire pit at Skjaermveien Barnehage (2009), Trondheim, Norway.* The Architectural Review *chose this for an award in its 2009 AR+D Emerging Architecture program. Courtesy of Haugen/Zohar Arkitekter.* (Plate 4)

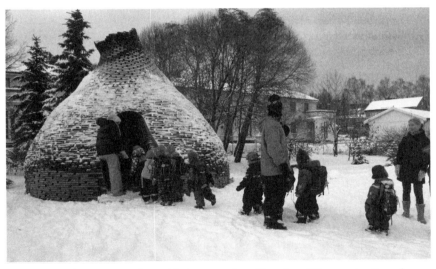

FIGURE 4.2 | *Haugen/Zohar Arkitekter, exterior of fire pit at Skjaermveien Barnehage (2009), Trondheim, Norway. These four-year-olds are coming to the hut to have their lunch. Author's photograph, 2012.*

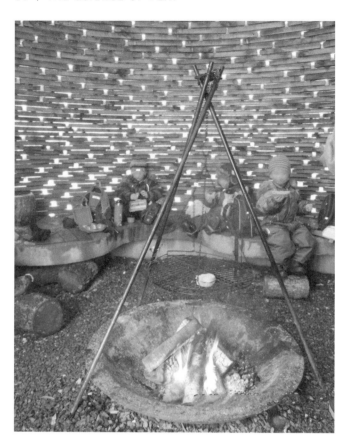

FIGURE 4.3
*Haugen/Zohar Arkitekter,
interior view of fire pit at
Skjermneien Barnehage (2009),
Trondheim, Norway. Author's
photograph, 2012.*

Aside from this "camplike" experience, nothing else that happens in the hut resembles anything that occurs on an American play yard. At noon, children put on their snowsuits and line up for the short trek to the "Fire Cabin." Each kid brings a lunch, frequently a cheese sandwich. They come into the hut, find a place to sit with their buddies, and take out their meal. Those who want to can toast their sandwiches on a grill suspended over the open fire pit. Teachers instruct children on how to execute this. They are always supervised, but children learn when they can approach the fire, how to make it work for them, how to retrieve the lunch, and when they should use the space just to sit and chat. Anyone observing them sees that these children are using restraint, following directions carefully, staying on task, and being diligent in their compliance. They are animatedly talking, sometimes even walking around in a very social setting.

On the other side of the world, American firm PWP Landscape Architecture (with Johnson Pilton Walker Architects) has been working on a project that tempts children to explore their relationship with water. Their Headland Park (due to open in 2015) is part of the enormous mixed-use (and often controversial) Barangaroo development west of the Sydney business district.[18] Industrial wharves filled the area in the nineteenth century, obscuring an early settlement by the Cadigal people. In the 1960s, container shipping yards dominated this land.

The Barangaroo project is set to revitalize this now-defunct industrial space by adding a cultural center and ample space for passive recreation as well as underground parking. Headland Park will be the primary green space in this newly reconstructed area. While there is no official playground, the designers see the entire park (almost six hectares, or fourteen acres) as a gathering spot for families. In addition to paths, grassy areas, and stairs (the site rises from sea level to over thirty-five feet), the designers have initiated the quarrying of the local Hawkesbury sandstone below the abandoned industrial areas. More than ten thousand stones have been unearthed and cut on site, thereby eliminating transportation costs and retaining an embedded resource. A new sandstone wall will follow the nineteenth-century shoreline.

There will be large sandstone blocks, partially submerged, along the new, extended shore. These "cascade" down to tidal pools. Families will have to be diligent in teaching their children how to interact with the water; kids will learn self-restraint and self-control while they experience a site that respects them and the traditional landscape. The "stepping stone" blocks will be playfully alluring; they evoke the small (and highly successful) concrete or wood steppingstones that Aldo van Eyck used on his tiny sites in Amsterdam in the mid-twentieth century.

Working Memory, Cognitive Flexibility

Working memory involves keeping a lot of information in the brain so that it can be continually rearranged and updated over time. Cognitive flexibility is the capacity to take account of different points of views and possibly be swayed by them; to see things in a new light; to reach novel conclusions. It also means possession of a supple outlook that is able to "take advantage of serendipity";[19] shift or switch between complex tasks;[20] and seize on unexpected opportunities.[21] Looked at together, working memory and cognitive flexibility support creativity. This has profound ramifications for playgrounds because we see that creativity is determined by how we approach a task. Working memory and cognitive flexibility set the groundwork for creativity to ignite. Once we understand that, we can recognize the futility of static equipment that advertises its ability to enhance the creativity of young folks.

When we think of handling and sorting through thoughts and juggling actual objects to produce something original, we are led back again to adventure playgrounds. Alex Gilliam, who runs Public Workshop ("a cheerleader for possibility") in Philadelphia, has built on the English adventure playground tradition and reinterpreted it. He secured several grants, including one from the Delaware Valley Green Building Council, to create a space in which young kids could use loose parts. Gilliam's approach has been to hire and rally teens. For one project, he hired high schoolers and college kids ("building heroes") to create a varied environment in Fairmount Park in Philadelphia.[22] They worked for most of summer 2013, erecting a series of ramps, folded planes, and elevated platforms. These often surround trees or tree stumps. Adjacent to the historic Smith Playhouse (known for a lovingly restored historic covered wood slide for all ages and an indoor traffic playground for toddlers), this adventure playground is an infrastructure where any child (starting about age eight) can move wood and learn to use power tools to add to the already built environment. Gilliam's two-pronged approach, anchored in first teaching older teens how to build, allows younger children to come later to the site and to experiment. It is a powerful model that has potential for being more acceptable to Americans because it seems more purposeful and focused than working solely with "junk."

Japan, currently a beacon for adventure play, has been doing its own versions since the 1970s. The translation of Lady Allen's *Planning for Play* in the late 1970s and United Nations declaration of the International Year of the Child in 1979 both may have sparked the movement.[23] There are now more than seventy adventure playgrounds ("playparks") that operate regularly (and more than one hundred others that function infrequently). Japanese adventure playgrounds are similar to others worldwide in that children are actively engaged with "loose parts" so that working memory and cognitive flexibility always underlie how they manipulate, arrange, rearrange, construct, and tear down constructions. These playparks seem to be especially strong in evoking their grass roots origins, employing "manipulative materials," and ensuring the long-term leadership of the play workers (called "play leaders").

Toyama Playpark in Shinjuku ward (where there are three other adventure playgrounds in the same district) is typical. In the late 1990s, parents in the neighborhood who wanted outdoor playgrounds got together. They petitioned the local government for support. Once the adults realized what an adventure playground was, they made that their goal. They focused on Toyama Park, even though it was then a haven for the homeless. After years of hard work and negotiation they achieved official status and began to re-ceive some funding from the ward in 2006. At that point they hired their first two full-time play leaders, who are paid partly by the Toyama parents' organization and partly by their ward.

Today, fifteen years after the first attempt to create something, several of the original parents (who now have grown children and sometimes have moved to different areas in the city) volunteer to keep their Toyama Playpark Organization running smoothly. The Japanese Adventure Play-ground Association reiterates this by saying that the playground is a citizen endeavor with a financial partnership between the citizens and the gov-ernment. Their success affirms the "ground up" approach that Amsterdam insisted on before Aldo van Eyck would design a neighborhood playground. The Japanese achievement is further validated by at least one family who bought a house adjacent to the park so that their three children could have immediate access to the facility.[24]

The layout of the Japanese adventure playground differs from those in the West. They are usually set within larger, long-established parks, which results in well-shaded sites. Many are open twenty-four hours a day and have no fencing. Children learn to use tools and understand the need to act responsibly. Older children who learn to saw, for instance, will commonly teach younger children how to handle the same tool. There is frequently an open fire; kids have to exercise self-control, and they have to learn when and what they can cook there. At Toyama, even preschoolers learn when to throw yams into the fire during an annual October festival.

Henegi Playpark (one of four adventure playgrounds in Setagaya ward) is the oldest adventure playground in Japan and presents the symbiosis be-tween an adventure playground and its host site. In this case, it is within the seventeen-acre Henegi Park, which has sports fields and a swimming pool. Since kids are free to go anywhere in the park, these young participants sometimes take their construction materials into the nearby woods, with a park official remarking that he has found an interesting construction far from the official playground. A permanent building, which opened recently within the playpark, underscores its role as a community resource and a place where parents delegate freedom to their children. A low structure with open sides, the new building is close to the entrance. It is a place for parents to stay and relax while their children use the site.

Children and play workers create high, fantastical buildings with old pieces of wood. Some are two and three stories high, a good indicator that working memory and cognitive flexibility have been activated. Children

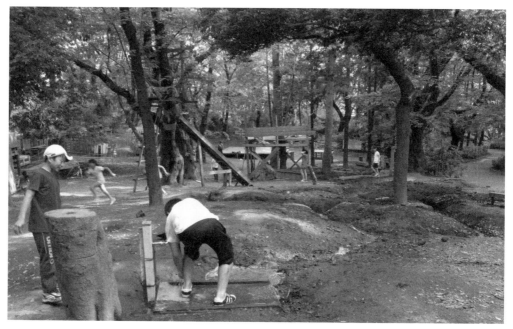

FIGURE 4.4 | *Henegi Playpark, Tokyo, Japan. This is the oldest adventure playground in Japan. Author's photograph, 2013.*

also dig deep ravines and then let water work its way down them. These "rivers" require planning (how much water will flow fast? How deep do they have to make the riverbank? What do they want to sail on these troughs?) Older kids in particular seem to relish getting muddy as they create water routes. Their pleasure is obvious as children — as well as those at Yume Park in Kawasaki, where the landscape is almost entirely mud — cavort in mud and stomp in their water routes. These stress-free settings may be useful medically, too. According to Adele Diamond, stress can alter the chemical balance (too much dopamine and norepinephrine) in the prefrontal cortex so that execution functions cannot be carried out properly.[25]

At Henegi and Toyama, play leaders perform in an extraordinary capacity: part teacher, part guide, part counselor. They assume a special role when a child gets hurt (not a common event, but something that everyone is aware can happen). At Henegi the motto is "Play freely under one's own responsibility," so the young people already know that they have to look inward for causes. If an accident occurs, the play leader works with the child to determine what went wrong. The objective is not to assign blame; it is to help the youngster see the mistake so as to avoid the same outcome in the future. This type of management is extremely potent and may explain

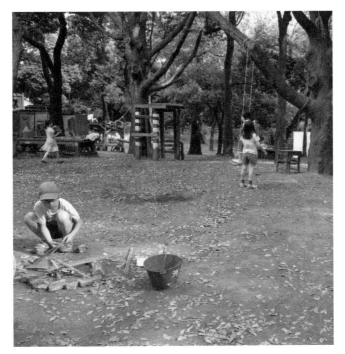

FIGURE 4.5
*Henegi Playpark, Tokyo. It is
not unusual for children to use
fires for cooking at Japanese
adventure playgrounds.
Author's photograph, 2013.*

why many of the former attendees (who age out in their midteens) will often come back to an adventure playground and seek out their favorite play leader. They look to them for direction and advice. Since many of the adventure playgrounds are in the less posh areas, the play leader provides a type of objective counseling that might not be available otherwise. A parallel and equally powerful phenomenon takes place in the United Kingdom, where adventure play continues at many locations. Children return to these sites and have lasting friendships with the play workers. There are instances where kids get older but never leave — moving from helper, to volunteer, to play worker.[26]

Leftover materials, in this case automobile and truck tires, dominate the Tire Park in Tokyo (Nishirokugo Koen in the Kanta section). This, too, was a grass-roots development started in the 1960s, which foretold our American craze for tire playgrounds of the 1970s, when advocates endorsed them for versatility and ready availability. The tires, after all, were free when taken from city dumps or car dealers.[27] In Tokyo, the menacing looking dragons or Michelin men became permanent and unalterable in the 1980s. For local kids, this park is a well-loved "obstacle course," perhaps named for so many of the tires that are permanently inserted in the ground and act as fencing for each of the construction areas. It does not appear to be run by the city,

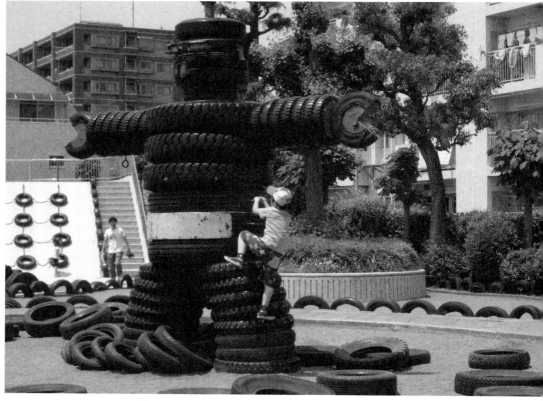

FIGURE 4.6 | *Nishirokugo Koen (Tire Park), Tokyo. Author's photograph, 2013.*

and it is unclear who maintains it; it straddles the notions of spontaneous playground and vernacular design.

The ability to use working memory or cognitive flexibility is not as great at the Tire Park as on an adventure playground but exists, nonetheless. There are opportunities to move tires anywhere that a child can place them, and to build something big. Kids can take them up on the wide slide; they can use them as the centerpiece of a sand creation. For kids who enjoy running, jumping, and swinging, there is some planning as to how and where to execute their moves. There is no shade, so children have to allocate their time judiciously in order to do the most construction in the shortest amount of time.

New Materials: Germany, United States

Not all adventure playgrounds rely on junk parts. Kolle 37, located in the Prenzlauer Berg, a neighborhood in Berlin, emphasizes the theme of "building" exclusively with wood.[28] The play space, explicitly meant to appeal to kids ages five to ten, also attracts a cohort of eleven- to twelve-year-olds who use it regularly. The building ethic at Kolle aspires to permanence and great height. Kids have to figure out how to achieve that. There are advisors who instruct kids on how to recognize that something is durable and how to continually test for strength. Some of the resulting "houses" are two and three stories high. Once a year, site managers take down the structures, allowing for continuing construction work in this area of densely packed construction. The safety record seems to be about the same as that of regular playgrounds.

Kolle 37, which prior to the unification of Berlin was in the eastern sector, began in the 1980s when teachers and artists used to haul a portable playground and art space around the city. The current permanent Kolle space dates to 1990. Fenced off from its immediate neighborhood, Kolle has views to the nearby shops and cafes so that it is not isolated. It is integrated into the neighborhood because anyone, even folks without kids, can come within its boundaries. It is part of an ensemble that includes a clubhouse and a larger park area that has a constructed hill, a site for bonfires, and a community garden. The area, which has a mix of ethnicities, has begun to gentrify, but there has been no threat to the existence of Kolle 37.

The site's costs are not extraordinary, but they are nonetheless somewhat high for adventure play. Kolle 37 buys most of its materials from construction companies, and neighbors provide a small amount of found materials. The local district (similar to an American borough or ward within a larger city) funds the cost of staff and some of the materials (about €120,000 [$150,000] per year), but Kolle 37 has to raise an additional €30,000 to €40,000 annually to support the site. The organization rents bikes; they charge for using their facilities for parties; they give special classes for schools or preschools.

Working memory plays a role, in that each child has to keep in mind what pieces and tools are available, and to suspend the impulse to do the easy or more temporary construction first if those actions would compromise the long-term success of each structure. Learning from their past experiences on the site, kids further galvanize their working memory by recalling where and how past failures occurred; they constantly have to consider which wood could be braced, and they have to keep that information closely at hand. If one piece doesn't succeed or is out of place, they must be flexible enough to change their plan and find another.

Playgrounds based on loose parts have even found their way into the United States, via the Rockwell Group, a multidisciplinary design firm led by David Rockwell.[29] Rockwell had observed that his two young children

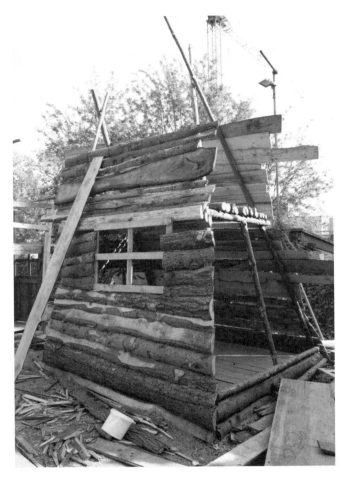

FIGURE 4.7
Kolle 37 "Abenteuerspielplatz,"
Adventure Playground, Berlin.
Courtesy of Nils Norman, 2006.
The Adventure Playground
and Playscape Archive.

were livelier and more creative in their apartment than they were outdoors. He noticed how they tore apart boxes and stacked cans at home but had few opportunities at their local playground to alter their environment. He began to believe that, as a designer, he could institute change within the city. He approached the New York City Department of Parks and Recreation at a particularly opportune moment: Parks Commissioner Adrian Benepe (now senior vice president and director of City Park Development at the Trust for Public Land), who had worked at positions within the Parks Department for most of his life, had witnessed the decline of interesting playgrounds. He had already committed his agency to bringing back sand to city playgrounds. His innovating spirit was spreading to those who worked for him, especially Assistant Commissioner Nancy Barthold.

New York City agreed to supply a site and, in partnership with the Lower Manhattan Development Corporation, to fund the construction costs. Additional funds, earmarked to keep families close to Ground Zero after 9/11, came from the federal Department of Housing and Urban Development; Rockwell Group worked pro bono. As they do for other city parks and playgrounds, the Parks Departments agreed to the maintenance and assumed the liability and daily costs. The site, Burling Slip, is a particularly intriguing one. It is within the historic South Street Seaport area, a nexus of tourist attraction, housing for the elderly, rent-controlled middle-class housing, and new high-end apartment houses.

Before beginning its design work, the Rockwell Group conducted serious research on play, playgrounds, and the history of the proposed site. They reached out to experts on children's development and sought as many views as possible. Roger Hart, of the Children's Environments Research Group of the City University of New York, was the strongest voice advocating that Rockwell consider loose parts and play workers. Rockwell Group committed its design team to creating something that would embrace those concepts. Perhaps more important for the future of the park, David Rockwell raised more than $1.8 million for an endowment for play workers. The idea of creating an endowment, and thereby ensuring the retention of play workers, appears to be a fresh concept in American park patronage.

The overall design of the permanent Imagination Playground is based on an elongated figure eight. This design effectively divides the site in half. One side is devoted to "dry" facilities, such as sand, a slide, and a long ramp that encourages running. The ramp provides many dark spaces for hiding. Nearby hoists, pulleys, and sand hark back to the site's marine history. The other half of the site is "wet," with a fountain and low amphitheater seating. Kids effortlessly bring sand and water together at both locations.

A small building that serves as both a comfort station and storage room anchors the area where the two loops meet. This modern shed stores the "loose parts." Rockwell Group designed buckets and wheelbarrows unique to the site. The iconic play items are bright blue loose parts in different geometric shapes designed in biodegradable foam. Play workers, now called play associates, make sure that blocks are brought outside and retired each day.[30] The associates are primarily there to make sure no activity gets out of hand. They gently coax parents to sit on the side and let the children join forces without parental direction.

Kids can work separately or together on building with the foam blocks. As the projects get bigger, the kids tend to become more collaborative. They all have to exercise restraint in not destroying the work before the group decides it is complete. They have to think quickly if something begins to

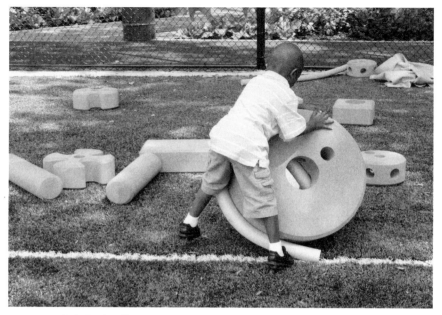

FIGURE 4.8 | *Rockwell Group, Imagination Playground in a Box (2010). This was an early play session to test the prototype for the foam blocks. Photograph by Robert S. Solomon, 2008.*

fall because it is not supported properly. And they have to draw on working memory to figure out what to add next. There is no single solution; only the children can decide when something is finished. The results indicate that kids find this approach liberating. They react vigorously and positively because they see endless possibilities, not unattainable perfection.[31] They also enact symbolic play, work out fantastic scripts, and talk to each other, all of which aid executive function.[32]

Buoyed by the success of the playground, Rockwell Group is now producing an "Imagination Playground in a Box." Parks departments and child-care facilities can now buy the waterproof foam blocks, which come in a self-contained bag, box, or cart. Rockwell is adding annually to the variety of shapes to keep the concept lively. The cost, under $10,000, is relatively low to change how a playground is perceived and used. Perhaps most meaningfully, the kit gives children the experience and presumed independence of an adventure playground. Author Nicholas Day, who has commented on the sameness of manufactured equipment, has noted that packaged loose parts may be the only way to rescue play from using only off-the-shelf equipment and to combat excessive litigation.[33]

Imagination Playground in a Box is now available in more than twenty countries, but anecdotes from New York City perhaps best indicate its impact. Assistant Commissioner Barthold notes that the city purchased two of the boxes when they first became available and has placed them in lower-income enclaves; they have added several more of them since. No blocks or boxes have been intentionally damaged or stolen. When she paid an early-morning visit to one of the sites, one with plenty of post and deck equipment, Barthold found a few kids sitting on the side. They had no desire to play on the ordinary equipment; instead they were content to sit quietly on the sidelines until the play worker arrived and brought out the blocks. Blocks, long associated with small geometric solids used in classrooms, have clearly been transformed into something more dynamic once the scale has been exploded and the site has been moved outdoors.

Noted landscape architect Ken Smith has also been thinking about loose parts and how they can improve public spaces. In 2009 he worked up a camouflage-based loose part system for a limited competition. Not currently in production, Smith's system suggests the power of loose parts to help children encounter critical EF functions, including keeping several things in mind before arranging or rearranging them, problem solving, and planning.[34]

For Smith, camouflage is a metaphor for hiding, concealing, and revealing. It's a concept that he has explored in previous projects, including the Orange County Great Park in Irvine, California, and a roof garden at the MoMA in New York. The program for the MoMA project, finished in 2006, called for materials that were lightweight, didn't require much or any water, were less than three feet high, and used white ballast that the museum already had in its possession. Smith devised a garden of man-made and stationary "loose parts," such as crushed glass, artificial boxwood trees and rocks, and recycled black rubber. The pattern was a vague reference to camouflage, since this was a partly concealed addition, one that masked the roof but can not be seen by most visitors.

Camouflage seems a suitable concept for kids, for whom hide-and-seek is still one of the most spontaneous and age-defying games, and who see the outdoors as conducive for these activities. In Smith's concept, which could have included a playhouse for storage, "CamousCAPES," pieces are not produced in camouflage colors or patterns; the camouflage is found in how kids (particularly those under five years) would maneuver them, how they could hide and nest some small pieces, or hide themselves under the large ones. The component pieces, which he envisioned in Roto Plastic or molded foam, would have been lightweight. Some pieces (CamouTOOLS)

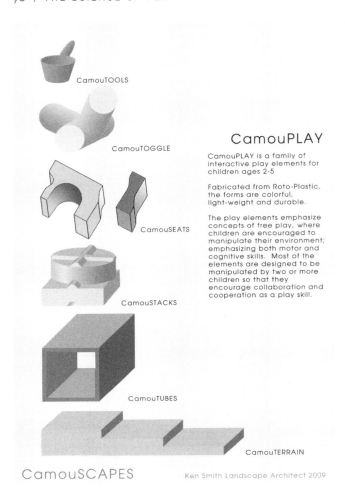

FIGURE 4.9

Ken Smith Landscape Architect, prototype for CamouPLAY (2008). Courtesy of Ken Smith Landscape Architect.

were variations on pails, shovels, and sand sifters. The CamouSTACKS elaborated on simple geometric shapes of circles, squares, and triangles. Fitted with ridges, these pieces were meant to stack high. The CamouTERRAIN pieces examined different "landscapes," such as stairs, ramps, and mounds. In the last case, Smith wanted these to be flipped over to be a "rocker" or boat. Both the STACKS and the TERRAIN pieces were large, in hopes of encouraging collaboration among children.

Smith envisions the production of the pieces in various colors, any number of which might be made available at a single site. Purchasers would "mix and match." Then kids, juggling all the possibilities in their minds, could construct structures that need thoughtful balancing and that could offer extensive hiding places. The abstraction here, and in Imagination Playground in a Box, encourages children to create their own scenarios on a large scale that are unusual in an open air setting. Very small preliminary studies hint at what we already suspect: that kids may be more physically active when they explore loose parts,[35] and that they may be more social in their activities.[36]

Sociodramatic Play

The role of sociodramatic play in heightening EF is not yet definitive, but it is nevertheless promising. A number of small studies support this hypothesis, but as yet there are no rigorous investigations with control groups, random assignment of participants, or other interventional assessments.[37] Still, we can cautiously and tentatively look at how it provides useful opportunities for kids in their cognitive development.

Fantasy play is at the heart of Vygostkian theory and is the centerpiece of a current Vygotsky-based curriculum, Tools of the Mind. Preliminary data shows that the Tools curriculum, which is based on taking a role, having to remember other people's roles, and then making adjustments as things play out, activates working memory, inhibitory control, and cognitive flexibility.[38] Its proponents say that Vygotsky believed that children (starting around age six) need play in order to "develop the creativity, self-regulation, and other underlying skills necessary for later development."[39] Fantasy has a logic in which children can describe the consequences of what happens within that pretense. But they also can see alternate consequences.[40]

Current science offers further clues as to why Tools (and fantasy, in general) might be welcome. One scientist, Silvia Bunge, speculates that Tools helps to develop the rostral lateral prefrontal cortex, the site of concentration and goal-setting. The Tools curriculum offers lots of choices, and Bunge notes that choice reflects motivation, which releases dopamine in the brain.[41] Additional data comes from researchers who have considered sociodramatic play in its own right. During sociodramatic play, young children verbalize what they are doing and therefore are able to self-regulate themselves and focus on a task.[42] Sharing pretend play lets small children experience shared emotions.[43] Kids who do role-playing learn how to see the point of view of others.[44]

It might appear difficult to offer role-playing in a public space, especially one without a play worker on hand to sustain dramatic play. The best way to design for sociodramatic play is to approach the project in a counterintuitive way. If a child wants to pretend to be a fireman, or a horseback rider, or a circus clown, then one might expect him to want to visit a space that looks like a firehouse or a ranch or a circus tent. In fact, literal equipment

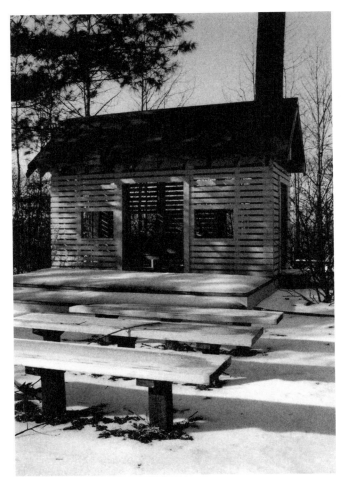

FIGURE 4.10
*Todd Rader + Amy Crews,
Playhouse for Elizabeth Morrow
Lower School playground (2007),
Englewood, New Jersey. Courtesy
of Todd Rader + Amy Crews
Architecture.*

(play boats, cars, or airplanes) tends to limit imagination. If we want kids to engage in fantasy, we have to give them the broadest notepad on which to write their own script. Abstraction, with only a hint of literal detail, is the most inclusive way to accommodate fantastical involvement.

An abstracted house is a simple and cost-effective way to bring pretend play to a public venue. Todd Rader + Amy Crews designed one (2007) for the Elizabeth Morrow School in Englewood, New Jersey. The school had commissioned the firm to design a master plan to link several buildings on their private campus. The school's administrators also wanted a fitness trail (not yet built) to be part of the scheme. Rader Crews took on those tasks and added a playhouse. They have avoided the pitfalls of most playhouses in the commercial catalogs, where pastel colors, cheap plastics, and gender specificity reign.

Their playhouse is elegant and spare, striking for its simplicity. It consists solely of a two-thirds scale shallow wood structure; only the carved animals on the front and side eave posts give a hint that it is intended for kids.[45] Wide spaces between wood slots allow for air and light. The composition is completed by a stage and picnic benches at the front. The colors of the house—mustard and deep red—are restrained. It is an abstraction: it is barely the sign for a house, which means that kids can pretend they are in a house; they could also imagine this to be a train station, a schoolhouse, or any other single-use building. The extra-wide and extra-high entrance means that it could be a firehouse or an airplane hangar. The shallow dimensions force children to interact in their fantastical activities. It also means that they have to navigate between tight "indoor" spaces and more expansive ones outside.

EF and Exercise

Data that links EF with exercise, especially aerobics, is beginning to look convincing. While we know that physical activity can positively affect the brain function of older adults "at the molecular, cellular systems and behavioral levels,"[46] we are beginning to understand that young children, especially those four to seven and eleven to thirteen, might also receive cognitive benefits from exercise.[47] According to cognitive neuroscience researcher Sarah Munro and her colleagues, "The brain does not recognize the same sharp division between cognitive and motor function that we impose in our thinking."[48] Aerobic running appears to improve the cognitive flexibility of eight- to twelve-year-olds.[49] It is possible that exercise is more effective if combined with carefully controlled activities, so that martial arts and yoga might be useful.[50] It is unclear at this point if organized sports, because they have not been studied, would provide the same benefits.[51]

Children who are aerobically fit are better at academics and cognitive control; they have "larger brain structures and more efficient brain function. . . . The performance differences are associated with neural differences, such that high-fit and lower-fit children show differences in the volume of the basal ganglia . . . as well as in event-related brain potential indices."[52] In an intriguing study, researchers applied this information to a simulated street crossing; they wanted to see if the fit children were more accomplished at street crossing under three different conditions: without distractions, while listening to music, and while talking on a hands-free phone. They found that the fit kids did better in all environments, although the authors cautioned that cell phones were a distraction to all children, including those

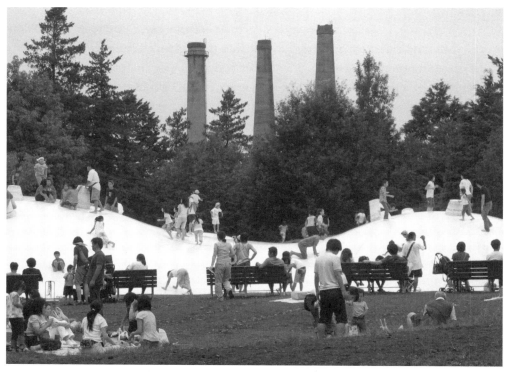

FIGURE 4.11 | *Takano Landscape Planning with Shiro Takahaski and Ogawatec tent company, Air Hill (1992), in Showa Kinen Park, Tokyo, Japan. Author's photograph, 2006.*

who were aerobically fit. These researchers speculate that, overall, fit kids may be better at multitasking.[53]

At a time when schools are pressured to devote more and more resources to academics and less to physical education, research indicates that programs that promote physical fitness improve not only physical health but cognitive health and academic achievement as well.[54] Adele Diamond concurs. She writes, "Improved physical fitness robustly improves cognitive and brain function, with prefrontal cortex and executive functions showing the greatest benefits."[55] The American government, which published "Physical Activity Guidelines for Americans" in 2008, calls for children and teens to get sixty minutes of physical activity each day. The government suggests that most of this activity be in the form of aerobic exercise, with muscle and bone-strengthening (high-impact) exercise making up the remainder of the time.[56] There is limited evidence that general physical activity increases when a child has a playground or schoolyard near home.[57]

These recent studies could positively affect planning for outdoor spaces. With this information, the confined activities on standard playground equipment seem all the more inadequate. It could be that we need to think of intense physical activities near or adjacent to the spaces where kids spend time. What might these intense physical activities look like? It may not be a crazy idea to include a dance stage near a playground or schoolyard. Creative dance and movement classes seem to enhance social gains.[58] Should there be running tracks near all playgrounds? Can we provide jump ropes and basketballs? What about martial arts, such as tae kwon do?[59]

One example in Japan may prove instructive. The "Bouncing Dome" (Takano Landscape Planning) at Showa Kinen Park is a site of intense physical activity. Young and old people try to outjump each other in height and endurance. Eventually, they fall down laughing. Then they start all over again. It appears to be group-oriented and more enticing than a trampoline. The dome is an air-filled membrane structure. Professor Shiro Takahashi (Tama Art University) holds a patent for the technology. Takano Landscape and Planning commissioned him to install a series of them (also called "air hills" or "pneumatic hillocks") at Showa Kinen Park, close to both Toshiko MacAdam's Rainbow Hammocks and Atsushi Kitagawara's and Fujiko Nakaya's Fog Forest. The commission, executed by Takano and tent company Ogawatec, was completed in 1992. It shows that shared spaces, among all age groups and family units, can be vibrant venues; it also confirms that aerobics can be practiced in areas that do not resemble traditional sports facilities. Children in Tokyo talk about going to play on the "marshmallows," a designation that implies springy resiliency and a special treat.

While we still don't know if aerobics will increase EF, the whole concept of EF is a promising way to evaluate play spaces. It offers new templates for how children manipulate and organize their environment and how we might construct ways for them to add planning and self-restraint to where they play. The next chapter adds friendship to this already dense mix of possibilities.

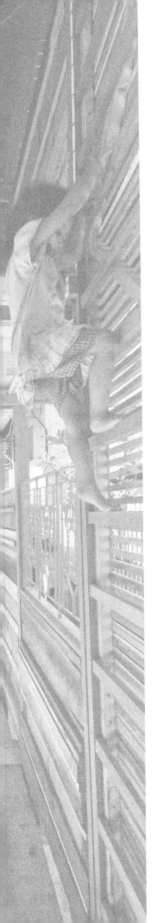

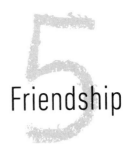

Friendship

FRIENDSHIPS SEEM LIKE SUCH AN obvious need. Kids require buddies for companionship, for exchanging fears and dreams, for learning to share and compromise, and for challenging each other physically and creatively. Friendships promote independence, fantasy play, and even understanding of other people. Children, who are naturally social, signal through friendship that they are ready to separate from parents. Having a friend is an early way to be independent of adults. In addition, having friends (more than acquaintances) fuels fantasy play, in which children immerse themselves in sustained and complex ways. Because of emotional attachments, friends — even young ones — try to negotiate and compromise to resolve differences.[1] And friendships have an effect on EF. Being sad or lonely impairs the development of EF capabilities.[2]

But friendship isn't always an obvious good. Children's friendships with nonrelated older adults, for instance, understandably raise wary parents' eyebrows. The things that kids like to do with their friends, too, can cause concern. Parents often have a particularly hard time acknowledging the positive contributions of rough-and-tumble (R&T) play for childhood development.

Effective playground design can not only facilitate risk taking, self-control, and problem solving but also can help to sustain friendships. Small parks, too, can enhance how kids get together with peers, and perhaps give them a chance to interact with people from other age groups, including the elderly. In rarer instances, public play areas can support teens, immigrant populations, and even survivors of natural disasters.

Recess and R&T

America does not have a recess policy; states or even individual principals can ignore it. In one state, legislation had to be enacted in 2012 to make sure the children received at least twenty minutes per day.[3] For five decades we have been trying to get kids to learn material — math and science in particular — at earlier ages than ever.[4] School districts, which often feel they have to choose between content and recess, often choose content because they believe it will get them closer to academic achievement. This trend has accelerated since the early 1990s.[5] Today, ubiquitous standardized testing, especially in the elementary grades, has fueled what educators see as a Hobson's choice.

Since the same era (the early 1990s), we have had increasing evidence that children learn better when they take frequent breaks. Studies from schools in Japan and Taiwan show that a break of ten minutes every hour improves learning outcomes.[6] Children (especially boys) are better able to concentrate after recess, and small kids need many breaks to learn.[7] Short breaks also provide greater social competence. The genesis of much of what we know about recess today comes from the "cognitive immaturity theory" that D. J. Bjorklund and B. L. Green first proposed in 1992. They argued that kids need breaks; otherwise they go into a cognitive overload that decreases learning.[8]

We are at present in a frightful cycle. Kids learn poorly because they don't get breaks; as a consequence, teachers feel that the students need homework to reinforce what they should be learning. The problem here is that long hours of homework appear to be counter productive.[9] The lack or limitation of recess, coupled with excessive homework, means that kids are getting a double whammy of exactly what they don't need. And more, both trends contribute to keeping children indoors. The American Academy of Pediatrics issued a stern policy report in 2012, which argues that we have to maintain "recess as an unstructured but supervised break that belongs to the child; that is a time for the child to make a personal choice between sedentary, physical, creative, or social options."[10] Physical education, while necessary, differs from recess.[11] When kids get to interact freely and without structures, "individuals learn to take other children's perspectives, comprehend and produce social signals, and inhibit their aggression."[12] To put it simply, recess supports peer interaction, especially in primary schools.[13]

Even when recess survives, schools most often ban R&T play. Chasing, wrestling, and other forms of vigorous, "rough" movements—the components of R&T—are healthful aspects of risk taking.[14] Most schools forbid it, but, counterintuitively, R&T play can lead to "regulating aggressive behavior."[15] This type of play fighting and chasing, especially for boys, may lead to games with rules such as tag rather than aggression.[16] Perhaps R&T would be more acceptable if it were explained as "energetic, competitive, body-contact play,"[17] which rarely becomes nasty or taunting.

Anthony Pellegrini, an expert on recess and R&T, has studied both for years in his educational psychology lab at the University of Minnesota. He sees R&T as a form of social interaction that sustains friendships (especially for boys) and allows physical communication to take place among peers.[18] Pellegrini is quite firm in his assessment that children know the difference between R&T and hostile behavior. Teasing, which can so easily look like bullying, may actually have an ability to enhance friendships until kids are close to eleven years old.[19] "Up to around eleven years," he writes, "most evidence suggests that the great majority of R&T is purely playful, and that when play fighting does turn into real fighting, this is due to a lack of social skills and not conscious manipulation."[20] It is easily sorted from aggression because participants laugh and smile; they are not angry or intent on causing harm.[21] R&T possibly promotes more intimate friendships.[22]

There are formidable cultural obstacles to allowing R&T play on playgrounds. In both the United States and Australia, teachers are fearful of getting sued if a child is injured,[23] and they tend to break up physical more than verbal altercations.[24] Americans have little tolerance for conflict or physical contact in play, whereas play workers in England are urged to stock materials for water fights and wrestling.[25] We tend to ignore the possibility that schoolyards could be a hospitable spot for R&T, where it can be monitored and thereby spare parents the worry that their children are in danger. Unlike aggression, which can take place anywhere, R&T could use a dedicated space.[26] It is preferable to have a place that is large and soft.[27] It may be that a unitary rubber surface, while a bore in most instances, is the ideal padding for R&T activities, especially since this an activity confined largely to the elementary school years.[28]

Two Yards: School and Club

Both recess and R&T have implications for public space. If we eliminate recess, then we also don't invest in schoolyards. As recent programs, such as PLANYC, have shown, playgrounds can become valuable public venues. How then can we make the schoolyard more fascinating to school kids and more welcoming to visitors from the community?

Katie Winter, the architect who designed the playground poles for Immaculate Conception School in the Bronx (chapter 3), has continually shown that a schoolyard can be inviting and versatile. Working largely for diocesan schools with minimal budgets, Winter has not let these constraints inhibit good design or friendly spaces. Consider, for instance, how she and fellow architect Charlie Kaplan transformed a parking lot into a playground for Resurrection School in New York in 2005. The client asked for artificial grass and a piece of climbing equipment. The designers saw to it that the

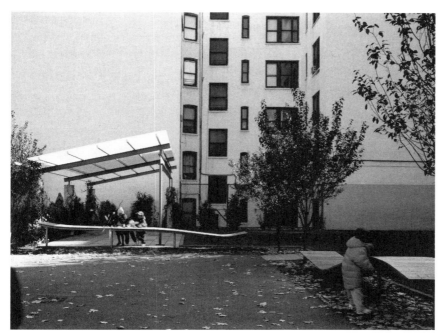

FIGURE 5.1 | *Katie Winter and Charlie Kaplan, Resurrection School (2005), Bronx, New York. Courtesy of Katie Winter Architecture.*

equipment, placed on a lower level, was adapted and placed close to a tree to allow for possible tree climbing. They followed the directive for artificial grass, then contrasted the flat horizontal plane with a bright yellow vertical one by painting the side of the building that borders the artificial turf. The openness of the space leaves lots of room for R&T and self-initiated games.

Along the perimeter, Winter and Kaplan added low rocks and benches, each unique, that they designed. They kept costs low by using off-the-shelf building supplies to create these handsome objects: standard galvanized pipe supports their centers and wood slats make up the actual undulating benches. Kids can invent games for these benches or use them as surfaces for rolling balls, hiding underneath, or piling onto as a group. The benches were intended for adults attending services at the adjoining church on Sundays. Adults can sit on them, but they are also high enough to rest cakes and coffee pots on.

The benches, rocks, and flat field mean that all of the grades (the original school has been replaced by a charter school) can have recess here at the same time. The abstract setting allows children to form their own age groupings: older kids can help younger ones. The playground is an excellent setting to support the ideal that Vygotsky called the "Zone of Proximal Development."

In Rotterdam, the firm 2012Architecten has applied some of the same principles of multiage cooperative use to a relatively low cost playground that promotes friendships and enrichment for an "at risk" immigrant population.[29] The board of a nonprofit "club," known as Kinderparadijs Meidoorn (Children's Paradise), asked 2012Architecten to renovate their old playground, which is adjacent to their indoor clubhouse. The architects developed a solution of creative reuse, including the repurposing of materials.

Children's Paradise (CP) is an unusual facility, one that is an inspiration for the way it has developed its curriculum and then allowed designers to translate their goals to the playground space. CP functions as an interventional program in the schools and then, again, at their "paradise" headquarters. Working in partnership with the schools and funded largely by the local government, CP stages workshops in the schools. They offer intensive study in the arts — dance, fine arts, music, theater — because they and the government believe that children who are not doing well in math or language skills will be helped by arts training. Although the program does not allude directly to self-control, it appears that that might be one of the things they are trying to introduce into the children's life. The after-school activities at CP's clubhouse reinforce and expand the workshops at school. Any child in the local schools can go there; sometimes a teacher will recommend that a child attend, and the child usually will. It is seen as a privilege: if children behave terribly on the playground, they are not allowed to come to the playground/club for two days, an indication of how important this site is to them.

CP puts emphasis on civility, how to learn to get along with peers, and how to develop long-term friendships. To that end, there are at least two adults on the playground. They allow free play (kids can come and go as they please, or as they have arranged with their parents) but also promote exercises that help the children to learn to obey rules and be polite and caring of each other. While the adult leaders guide the kids, they also let them set the rules and parameters.

Since CP accommodates children four to twelve years of age, the playground had to be able to appeal to differing age ranges. The budget was €250,000 (approximately $340,000), a budget that usually permits the purchase of just a few off-the-shelf pieces. (For comparison, the six pieces of equipment and rubber surfacing at Sue Bierman Park playground in San Francisco had a price tag of more than $700,000, for which a local friends group had to raise funds). All parties at CP — the board, the club, and the

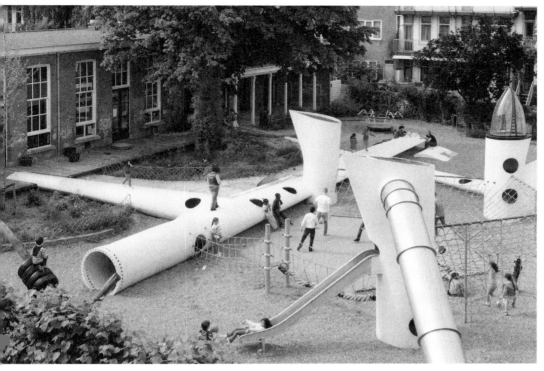

FIGURE 5.2 | *2012Architecten (now Superuse Studios), playground (2009), Rotterdam, Netherlands. The most vigorous activity is in the panna pitch; calmer areas are where blades blend into or near the clubhouse. Photograph by and courtesy of Denis Guzzo.*

architects — wanted an unusual play space, one that would challenge the kids to invent their own play.

For Césare Peeren, the head designer for 2012Architecten and the person who had researched playgrounds with his son, the task was to complement the social goals while simultaneously respecting the scale and composition of the neighborhood. This is an area of low, nineteenth-century worker houses in the northern part of Rotterdam, one of the few parts of the city not bombed during World War II. The area is ethnically and economically diverse.

Peeren chose discarded wind turbine blades from Dutch windmills as the primary building material and organizing principle for the playground, dubbed Wikado. The blades, which stay in service for only ten to fifteen years, are readily available. The only cost in acquiring them is the expense of trucking them from the countryside to the city. Using them was a clever environmental decision, too. Between twenty and forty-five thousand discarded blades are burned each year in the Netherlands, so the reuse has reduced toxic emissions. Repurposed to a playground, the blades need a fresh coat of paint every three or four years but are otherwise maintenance-free.

A small alleyway is the access route from the street to both the playground and the clubhouse. It is the first place where it is possible to see a blade, a harbinger of things to come. In this case, it is half buried in the sand and stone ground but directs the visitor to the large central space. Inside the playground, two additional blades "melt" into or just up to the clubhouse. This extends the playful activities into the building, a gesture that is appreciated in a country with short winter days, although the children are encouraged to play outdoors unless it is very wet. For the central play area, Peeren placed all five turbine wings, each thirty-five meters (over one hundred feet) long, into a loose overlapping grid. He scattered them about in a way meant to resemble the childhood game of pick-up-sticks. Holes of 1.4 meters diameter (less than four and a half feet) were cut into the blades at various locations to give the kids a way to climb through and investigate each interior. By cutting holes, the architects supported "hide and seek," a favorite game that can be played within. They also provided intimate spaces for two or three kids who want some relaxing time sitting together.

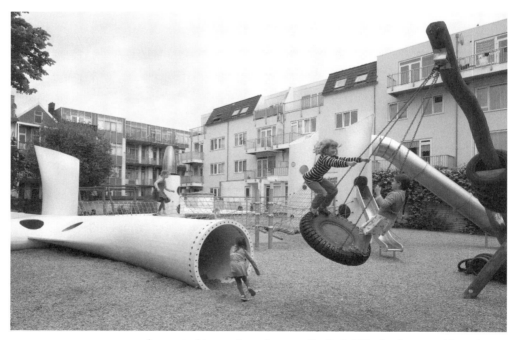

FIGURE 5.3 | *2012Architecten (now Superuse Studios), Wikado playground (2009), Rotterdam, Netherlands. Photograph by and courtesy of Denis Guzzo. (Plate 5)*

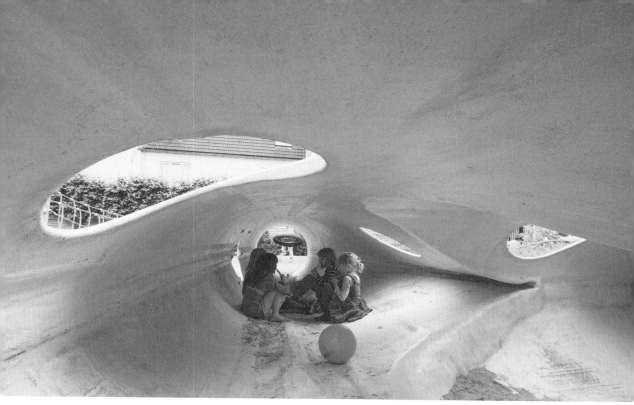

FIGURE 5.4 | *2012Architecten (now Superuse Studios), Wikado playground (2009), Rotterdam, Netherlands. The interior of the blade is good for quiet moments. Photograph by and courtesy of Denis Guzzo.*

In addition to the enclosed spaces created by the wind turbine blades, Peeren added four towers, thereby extending the playground into a vertical zone that children can climb. One of these allows kids to pump water that then flows through holes and down the blades. Another is a climbing tower with an observation post; two F16 cockpit covers rest over the top. A third provides access to a slide, extended and reused from the old playground. The fourth tower offers interior climbing. Together, the four towers enclose a panna pitch, a local version of street football.

2012Architecten did a fine job of integrating the different ways that children of varying ages approach a playground and need to occupy the same space simultaneously. By using the towers to suspend a panna net, the designers effectively delineated the more active sectors from the more passive ones. Older children, especially boys, head to the panna area and the towers. Younger kids will gravitate to a merry-go-round and the swings. The peaceful areas — near the sand and some stripped dead trees and in the interior space of the blades — are important for escape in a space that has twenty to thirty active children at a time.

Friendly Places

In addition to schoolyards and club spaces, public settings should also have high priority as places where kids — and adults — can hang out. All offer children opportunities to interact and form lasting bonds.[30] The importance of these experiences intensifies as kids get older. Educational psychologists who study adolescents tell us that when kids enter middle school, they rely more than before "on friends for companionship, intimacy, and support."[31]

Extensive public settings in Rotterdam and Tokyo present us with some of the best paradigms of places that encourage those interactions, where young people especially can settle their own disputes and gain some insights into the thinking of peers. In Rotterdam, designer and historian Liane Lefaivre takes inspiration from the small, postwar playgrounds — "extended polycentric network" — that filled unused space in Amsterdam after World War II (Chapter 2).[32] She has been using the same principle, which she calls PIP, for Polycentric, Interstitial, Participatory Public Space, in designs for the Oude Westen and Hoogvliet sections of Rotterdam. Many of the residents in these neighborhoods are poor immigrants; the availability of nearby playgrounds means that neighbors feel more comfortable being in an open setting and that children can easily move, usually with their friends, from one site to another among the dense web of play spaces.

Tokyo, perhaps unwittingly following the van Eyck model, has its own "web" in each neighborhood; these are small parks that happen to have a piece or two of playground equipment or a sandbox. The idea of a profusion of parks has existed in Japan for more than thirty years. In the early 1980s, the mayor of Tokyo bragged about the proliferation of parks and their easy availability; he claimed that each child had a playground nearby. Scholar Joy Hendry believes that is still accurate, and that most Tokyo children live within a hundred meters (three hundred feet) of a playground.[33] It is easy (and very common) to be able to walk to several within a few minutes' time, especially given the density of Tokyo (and the small living quarters from which everyone is happy to retreat). A playground could be on the main shopping street; it could be off in a separate corner. The ready availability of these playgrounds means that private day care establishments can take advantage of them: frequently kids walk (two-by-two or holding onto a rope) through the neighborhood shopping street several times a day to get to the park.

At first glance, these mini parks look a bit unkempt and a bit too minimal, possibly uninviting. The ground cover is usually dirt, the entrances do not

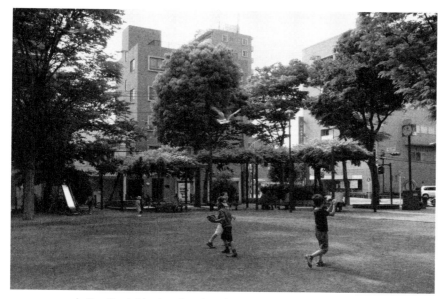

FIGURE 5.5 | *Small neighborhood park, Tokyo, Japan. This park has shaded area for adults, a small amount of equipment for children, a large empty space for sports or games, and the ubiquitous clock. Author's photograph, 2013.*

have gates, and there is no perimeter fencing. The swings or climber, which are usually antiquated, tend to have some springy material underneath; low bars often surround the swings in order to protect younger children who walk by, an efficient remedy that improves on our concept of "use zone." Some greenery, seating, a water fountain and a spigot, and a clock are common characteristics to most of these parks.[34]

It is easy to dismiss these urban slots as uninspiring, boring. To do that would be to miss the powerful role that these miniparks have in each neighborhood and in the well-being of local residents. There is an audio system; at 7:00 each morning it blasts out the government's workout program for seniors. Elders could also hear it on a radio at home, but it becomes a social (and more enjoyable) event when they do their movement exercises together. The benches, in addition to providing a resting place, frequently have information on how these seating areas can be used as exercise stations throughout the day. Young children come with caregivers in the later morning or afternoon.

When parents bring preschoolers to these parks, they teach them how to ask for a turn on the swing or some other apparatus. Kids and adults use *Janken* (a Japanese version of rock, paper, scissors) to settle disputes.[35] Robert Aspinall, who teaches at Shiga University and takes his own six-year-old

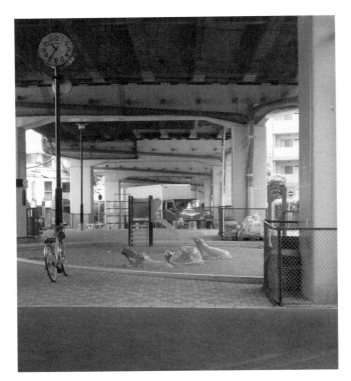

FIGURE 5.6

Small neighborhood park, Tokyo, Japan. This park was shoehorned into leftover space beneath a highway. Author's photograph, 2013.

son to parks in another Japanese city, Nagoya, has found that these "are very friendly places where parents encourage their children to play with other children. Parents often use the word *tomodachi* (friend) for another child they have only just met."[36]

The Tokyo parks foster a sense of community, an extension of *Uchi*, where mutual cooperation occurs. Chris Berthelsen's calculation of the street, as a place where kids learn to navigate with traffic and other individuals, carries over to the playground. Young children, teens, older folks, drunks, office workers taking a break or eating lunch, might all be there together. Everyone has some tolerance for others. Infrequently, a park will be shoehorned into a leftover spot under a highway or bridge. In that instance, there might be just a few pieces of equipment without benches or greenery, but there is still a clock. There might also be some homeless people, but that does not make the site unsavory for children.

There is an underlying attitude of personal responsibility and a pervading sense that looking after the good of all children is a collective task. There are no play rangers or play workers, yet it is not uncommon for a six-year-old child in Tokyo to go to the playground by himself. It is not just that Tokyo is considered a safe city, which it is, but that children are respected as responsible young folks. Kids can meet up with friends, travel alone or in packs, then branch out to other play spaces. They can begin to act independently, developing friendships in the quiet areas where they can chat or exchange cherished trinkets. When the park clock chimes at the end of the day (5:00 p.m.), children know that it is time to return home for supper.[37]

The spirit of contemporary Japanese playgrounds invokes an unlikely comparison. In 1961, urban advocate Jane Jacobs wrote about her life in the 1950s on Bethune Street in New York City's Greenwich Village. Jacobs wrote about the vitality of the life of the street, a place where people watched out for each other in a kind and generous way. Kids had great latitude to play in the neighborhood. American urban planners have been trying to capture that sense of community spirit and awareness for decades. It is ironic that it exists, not in America, but in Tokyo.

Older Adults in Spaces for Young Kids

There is some evidence that strong relationships between young children and older adults can have a positive effect on the lives of kids. The younger generation learns to respect the elderly, rather than fear them; as a consequence, teens become aware of their own mortality and act more cautiously when it comes to negative risk taking (for example, drugs, alcohol) as they get older.[38] The documenting of relationships between younger children and their grandparents is much more extensive and conclusive. Positive outcomes include reduced symptoms of depression and better overall psychological well-being.[39]

Most of the research on intergenerational activities has centered on programs that bring young and old together, usually in an institutional setting. In some cases the young and the old share facilities, such as a day care center in a home for the elderly. While there is still very little attention to how young and old could use the same outdoor spaces, some playground stakeholders are beginning to consider the question. In 2009, the manufacturer Lappset sponsored an "International Design Competition for 3 Generations." The winner, Georgian Tengiz Alaverdashvili (from Tbilisi), designed a low rising hill with extensive benches. It is unlikely that it will be put into production but this type of competition may just be starting, and it is possible that later versions will lead to built designs.

For the present, it is useful to think of how intergenerational space can exist as an integrated public entity. In Israel, Avi Laiser's "Real Estate" in the city of Bat Yam has an enormous sign that proclaims: "the REAL estate." Laiser's piece, with its funny play on words, may give a hint of an irreverent view of what public space can accomplish.[40] Laiser, an American-trained architect (MArch, SciArc) who returned to his native Israel in 2000, began the installation as an art project. Together with his wife, the dancer Dana Hirsch Laiser, the architect submitted an idea to Bat Yam's International Biennale of Landscape Urbanism (2008). Curators gave them the nod, even before they had a site, to create one of the "temporary private spaces" that would help to define the event.

Laiser, who also develops high-rise apartments, knows the value of public space as a way to enhance property values in an up-and-coming community. In order to have the greatest impact, the couple therefore chose a location that, at first glance, would appear to be problematic. It was literally a dump, a leftover space on the side of an eighteen-foot-high (six-meter) noise barrier at the side of the congested Ayalon Highway. Neighbors had used the plot to abandon mattresses and toasters, or as a dog park or place to buy or sell drugs. The only positive thing happening there was the burning of bonfires during the Jewish holiday of Lag B'Omer each spring.

The Laisers saw the site differently. They were interested in edge conditions and the dichotomy between private and public spaces. Avi Laiser points out, for example, that we "privatize" public space for a short moment when we sit on a bench or put up an umbrella at the beach. Their goal, in short, was to reclaim a space that would become like "a home outside." The organizing city, Bat Yam, was supportive of these ideas because their municipality is densely populated and diverse, including a large Vietnamese population.

The Laisers designed a structure, not unlike a ski slope, that starts flat on the ground and then rises dramatically as it goes along the wall of the noise barrier. The structure includes both hard and soft materials. Grass at the edges encourages older people to sit, but the main seating area comprises free-form shapes that have been sunk into the rigid surface covering. Lined with wood, these abstracted forms have interior ledges. The Laisers found that there is a good mix of ages but that teens are drawn to the enclosed, well-defined "depressions" close to the ground. Because of the ledges, these deeply cut "nooks" can accommodate large and small groups of friends. These are comfortable places, partially hidden and partially obvious, in which teens can adapt the "edge" to be their new "center." At first, kids flooded these intimate gathering spaces; now adults come to hang out, too.

With Avi Laiser acting as general contractor, the final price was modest, about 300,000 shekels ($185,000). The Biennale paid for construction costs;

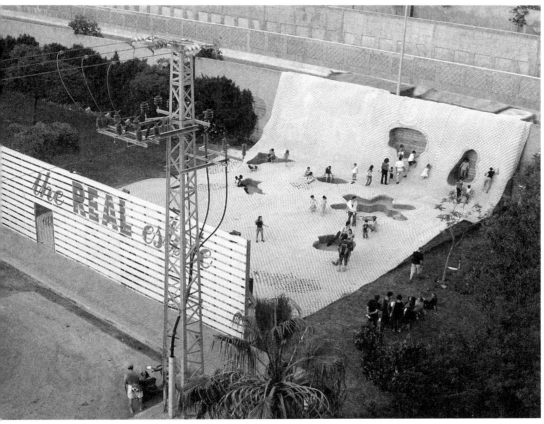

FIGURE 5.7 | *Avi Laiser and Dana Hirsch Laiser, The REAL estate (2008), Bat Yam, Israel. Courtesy of Laiser Architecture. Photograph by Avi Laiser.*

the city maintains the site. This manmade park is open twenty-four hours a day, thereby defying a trend in Israel (and so many other countries) to lock down spaces at night.

Teen-Places

Teens represent a special difficulty because they often want to be away from everyone else. One study in Finland shows that young teens were likely to visit favorite places with their peers; often their parents did not even know where these places were.[41] While we have already seen that they might be drawn to thrilling activities, they are also seeking both activity and quieter places, maybe even updated versions of "hiding."

BASE, the same landscape architects who designed the playground in Belleville Park in Paris (Chapter 2), have a new project: Sergent Blandan Park in Lyon.[42] They expand their ideas about identity and risk taking.

It is specifically geared to teenagers, although it could be used by those younger or older. The clients—the city and the surrounding region (both of which have a reputation for cutting-edge concepts in their public buildings)—believed that an abandoned army base could become an urban oasis of twenty hectares (fifty acres). BASE won a competition for this project, now one of the largest recreational redevelopment efforts in Europe. The total project cost will be €20 million ($27 million). The complex program includes integrating nineteenth-century defensive walls and fortifications, a fifteenth-century castle, and some twentieth-century buildings into a single public park. Some ruined buildings have been retained as nature spaces where vegetation sprouts among remains of construction.

BASE set aside the old parade ground for the active play area. The large scope of the space means that there will be other areas for quiet interaction. For the dedicated play space, BASE has designed an elaborate oak structure. Where the playground at Belleville Park is steep and confined by the original site, this play space is very wide as well as high. As at Belleville, kids can hoist themselves up and enter "unexplored" territory; sometimes they hoist but cannot go any farther. Other times, they enter an immense shallow wood structure with different levels, large and small areas, and dead ends. The architects hope to achieve spaces, like a labyrinth, where children don't always know where they are going.[43] They have to find their way, by trial and error, until they reach long slides to the exterior. Gravel pits and benches at the bottom of each of these enclosed slides ensure that teens will have a place to rest and hang out before they try the ascent again.

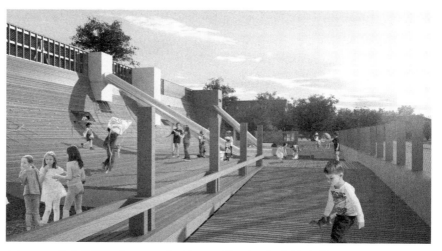

FIGURE 5.8 | *BASE, playground at Sergent Blandan Park (digital image, 2013), Lyon, France. Courtesy of BASE.*

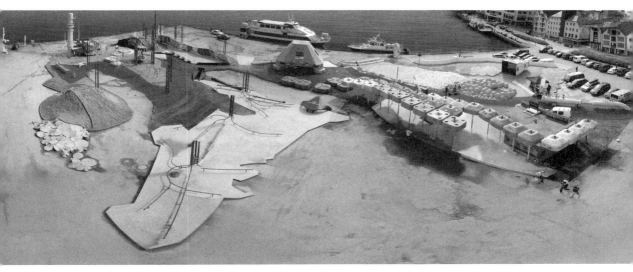

FIGURE 5.9 | *Helen & Hard, Geopark (2008), Stavanger, Norway. Courtesy of Helen & Hard. Photograph by Emile Ashley. (Plate 6)*

Another approach to enticing adolescents into public spaces is to provide areas where they can enjoy each other and in which they can gather and show off. Norwegian architects Helen & Hard saw such a need in their hometown of Stavanger.[44] A prosperous small city at the administrative hub of the booming oil industry, Stavanger lacked a gathering spot for teens. Helen & Hard took it upon themselves to address that in 2008 in preparation for Stavanger's becoming the European Capital of Culture. Their creation, Geopark, repurposes leftover objects from exploration at the enormous Troll oil field in the North Sea. They have organized the terrain to express the geological layers of the oil site. By using materials that are no longer useful, Helen & Hard have alluded to local industry at the same time that they have established an industrial vernacular, a definite "place" that reflects the economic prosperity of the city as well as its industrial waste.

Helen & Hard created an "other worldly" landscape that abuts the harbor and is unfenced. Anchors and buoys provide sheltered seating for quiet times. There is also the chance to be active in resourceful ways. Some of the found objects are quite high; low pipes sprawl out in several directions. Teens are free to do whatever they choose. All of these oil industry implements are so strange to daily life that they invite teens to come up with new ways to employ them. They might dare each other to see who can climb the high poles. A section of immovable balls has become a place to run and jump. These red balls also allow for teen exhibitionism in the form of back flips, tumbling, and crazy acrobatics. It is possible that there is an oral history developing, too, in which teens might continually embroider and discuss the heroic feats they accomplish here. That type of self-propelled competitive engagement will have kids wanting to return for a very long time. They are also drawn to skateboarding and many surfaces for graffiti, both of which are acceptable here. These activities have already transformed the overall look of the site. Spray-painted graffiti fits comfortably with the city's annual NuArt Festival that highlights street art. The park, which never closes, is enticing in the summer when days are long.

A Place of Refuge

In 2000, Art for the World, an NGO associated with the UN Department of Public Information, sponsored an exhibition and accompanying program to bring artists (including architects) into the design of toys and playgrounds for refugee children. The first results were powerful responses to often tragic existences. Whereas the focus of that exhibit was children caught in political turmoil, natural tragedy has created a different type of necessity in Japan. Following the devastating earthquake and tsunami in 2011 more than sixty cities and villages were destroyed, and the long-term outlook is for a slow recovery. Children and adults may be living in temporary housing for several years.

Tokyo architect Toyo Ito, the 2013 Pritzker Prize Laureate, became an activist over the issue of reducing some of the misery. Shortly after the damage occurred, he organized a group of peers (including Kengo Kuma and Kazuyo Scjiima) and, working with the Japan Foundation, established the Home-for-All Project. Their objective — largely achieved within a year — was to design and build community gathering centers in areas where the people were living with great difficulty. Five firms finished five centers in less than a year.

Once those projects were launched, Ito turned to the plight of children. Realizing that the surviving children needed stability in their lives, he invited a former student, Maki Onishi, to create a space dedicated to them.[45] Onishi worked in the temporary town of Greentown Yamoto in Higashi Matsushima on a play project that the local residents manage and supervise. She devised three small houses, each with a distinctive roof of either a dome, a pyramid, or a spire. These houses sit on a low platform, the one element that draws them together. One is a Home of Table, which provides a place for "hanging out," doing craft projects; another is a Home of Wood Stove for cooking or warming; and there is a Home of Theater for impromptu performances. Together, these are meant to be a small village where young people can "get together, exchange their ideas and achieve heart-to-heart relationship."

Onishi has shown that dire circumstances can inspire architectural help and uncompromised design. It is possible to build quickly and efficiently. The spaces, small and inviting, provide many chances for friendships to develop and be sustained.

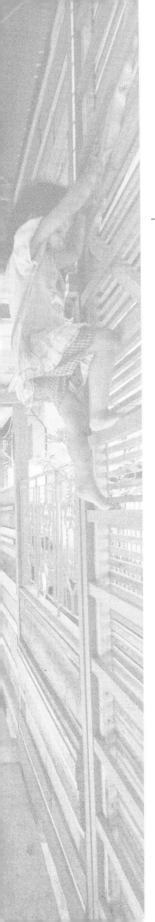

Nature and Exploration

"NATURE" AND "EXPLORATION" seem to be a well-matched pair that highlight two of the strongest themes in contemporary design for play. "Natural playgrounds" have become a rallying cry, a backlash against manufactured equipment, in the United States and parts of Western Europe. Proponents proclaim the value of nature in fostering exploration. They maintain that natural spaces allow kids to gain independence, to learn to cooperate, and to achieve greater cognitive and emotional control. Advocates cite nature as a remedy to mitigate the constraints of learning disabilities or abject poverty.

It is no longer uncommon for a parks department to issue a request for qualifications (RFQ) which states that they are looking only for designers of equipment-free, natural playgrounds.[1] Parents and administrators, eager to avoid mundane playgrounds and motivated by the publicity about nature playgrounds, have latched on to natural playgrounds as the best—and sometimes only—option. The localvore movement, with its calls for sustainability and a sense of place, has fueled the trend. There is an underlying hope that children who are exposed to nature will grow into adults who want to protect the environment.[2]

Given the activity and hype, this is a fine moment to take a look at the natural playground movement, assess it, and identify both its best practices and its shortcomings.

Assessing Nature Play

It is refreshing that adults are no longer satisfied with the status quo. Play patrons are seeking solutions that will occupy kids more successfully than does static equipment; they are looking for opportunities for exploration and experimentation. Nature does offer an affordable way to challenge kids with variety, variability, and unpredictability. There is no right or wrong when kids play in a natural setting; such venues often provide chances for risk, mastery, planning, and problem solving. Dirt, in addition to being hugely entertaining (kids might even perceive it as playing somewhere "naughty" if they have not been acculturated to avoid it), can bring children of different ages together. It is an especially healthful material with which to boost the immune systems of young children.

Nature is perfect for little kids because it is not static. Once babies become toddlers, they need to experience different surfaces to increase their balance skills. Nature offers a chance to encounter the irregular and the unexpected. Sand piles and water buckets make sense and provide natural materials for toddlers; a wider environment of trees, bushes, streams, and rocks will, of course, provide lively spaces for older children. Nature play can also give young children a reprieve from overzealous parents and educators who push reading and writing too early in a child's life. Forest Schools, developed in Scandinavia in the 1950s and then in the United Kingdom since the early 1990s, might provide an interesting alternative. Children regularly go to densely wooded areas where there are free play and preplanned activities, and where they can master "small achievable tasks."[3]

The downside, which we cannot ignore, is that there are a few troubling aspects to the nature movement. In spite of absolutist rhetoric from advocates, natural playgrounds do not have a lock on exploration, sustainability, or sense of "place." We have already seen that some pieces, such as Haugen/Zohar's cube or their fire pit, are made sustainable by repurposing materials that would otherwise have created industrial waste. The playground at Belleville Park (BASE), the PlayStreet at Potgieterstraat (Carve), and the Children's Paradise (2012Architecten) are just three examples of how a well-designed playground can emerge from both cultural values and manmade materials to create a unique individuality and locale.

Projects have sprung up that embrace the message, but not the spirit, of nature play. The term "nature play" is being used indiscriminately. Some designers are calling for the usual equipment but adding a few bushes or trees in the hope that these will count as "natural" designs. Play advocate and author Tim Gill has labeled the practice as "insulting [to] our intelligence and aesthetic sense."[4] Some manufacturers, missing the point that a natural playground has a life and death, are creating concrete logs and saying that they represent a durable "natural play" area. One Florida town used a $200,000 privately funded grant to create a park (named for a local early-twentieth-century naturalist!) that has imitation trees; faux tree trunks sit on either side of a low slide. There are "swings hanging from pretend tree trunks . . . big model ant hill to climb through . . . butterflies and caterpillars to ride on [and] . . . a mushroom table."[5] Since nothing is living, there are posted signs that have information ("educational messages") about nature.

Sometimes "natural playground" has become a meaningless title for a space that is just as regimented as a traditional playground. Some adults—and it is often unclear whether the pushback is coming from administrators, parents, or both—are often reluctant to accept the unpredictability that nature should provide. A "Natural Playscape" in Iowa, for example, has set rules that controvert the variability, messiness, freedom, and openendedness of nature play that the park's design should encourage. A sign that would be risible in Scandinavia—where kids experience nature by themselves and with little supervision or rule—tells children how to behave. The sign, which reveals the imprint of an insurance-conscious municipality, says that children should be at least five years old to play there; they should not climb trees or rocks nor pick flowers or feed the animals; they must wear shoes; their parents should supervise them at all times; and they should be careful when the "playscape" is wet.[6] So much for "nature play."

Equally disturbing is the way that natural playground proponents, especially those in North America, extol preliminary scientific studies. They present tentative and hypothetical conclusions as if they were absolute facts. They laud nature play, for instance, as a panacea for social and behavioral problems. While there is some evidence that children are more involved with what they are doing when they play in a natural environment,[7] most of the evidence is not conclusive.

We just don't know yet if nature—undiluted, unaltered—has mythical powers on its own. Today's promoters of natural playgrounds are caught in a game that resembles that old standard, "telephone." (Maybe today we could call it "Internet.") Someone says something to someone else, who then passes it on. As the information makes the rounds of successive individuals, the message changes until it reaches a point at which it is no longer recognizable. In the case of natural playgrounds, preliminary research with tentative conclusions circulates until it emerges as absolute "fact"; limited findings morph into hard truths.

The documentation (much of which is cited by those who want to make the connection between nature play and improved lives) shows something more subtle, vague, and responsible. The most visible researchers, Frances Kuo and Andrea Faber Taylor, are frequently quoted because of their investigation of nature as a way to manage ADHD. Proponents of nature play represent their work as an unabashed endorsement of nature's benefits. A closer look shows that their findings are preliminary and not definitive. They have written that their evidence, while encouraging, will not be conclusive without broader, randomized, controlled, and larger studies. They state, "With a few exceptions, most of the studies have methodological weaknesses that need to be addressed through future research."[8] They are encouraged that the early results can now justify broader and deeper investigations. There was little press attention when Taylor and Kuo recently wrote responsibly that it is "unresolved" whether "routinely experienced greenspaces have systemic effects on children's ADHD symptoms."[9] And yet, it is not uncommon to see their tempered views transformed into statements that claim that the experience of nature can alleviate ADHD.

There are other guarded views about how the public receives and transmits information about nature. The University of Essex conducted a review of literature on "large natural habitat and wilderness experience" for the Wilderness Foundation. Describing the limitations of their efforts, they wrote that more than 80 percent of the literature was qualitative or descriptive; the number of studies that purported to be quantitative was about 14 percent, but often the cited samples had fewer than thirty people and no control group.[10]

Another able researcher in the field of nature and its impact on adults puts it this way, "What seems evident — whether focusing on relatively ordinary and familiar natural settings during middle childhood or more challenging and undisturbed environments in adolescence — is that direct experience of nature plays a significant, vital, and perhaps irreplaceable role in affective, cognitive, and evaluative development." But he also concludes that "more study, of course, is needed before this conclusion can be confidently accepted."[11]

Is Nature the Best Way to Simulate Nature?

We Americans have been trying to simulate or incorporate nature into playgrounds for more than five decades. It is essential to remember, especially for those adults who bemoan the fact that their kids don't play in dirt or roll logs across the ground, that nature was an undercurrent that inspired innovative playgrounds of the 1960s and 1970s. M. Paul Friedberg, one of the early advocates for linking playground elements together, believed that playgrounds should allow urban kids to have the gratifications of traipsing through nature. His approach was to give wood and stone, water, and sand to New York City kids to simulate the types of unexpected encounters they would have if they were living in upstate New York and playing in a local stream. Certainly, jumping from one wood piece to another, scaling up a granite mound, or digging into deep sand must have been fairly good substitutes. Some of the smaller spaces to hide would have shown how kids in the wild create their own intimate environments.

Landscape architect Robin Moore and educator Herbert Wong took an even more literal approach to nature during the 1970s. They transformed a macadam school playground into the "Environmental Yard" at Washington Elementary School in Berkeley, California. It took a decade of marshaling aid from parents and students to complete the metamorphosis. Children were enthusiastic beneficiaries; they could make choices, test their own limits, even fail in a lush environment of trees, plants, and water.[12] It is worth recalling, however, that even the Environmental Yard was not a totally natural space; the originators provided sections for quiet group meetings, kickball and basketball, and even climbing equipment.[13]

There is a cautionary tale here. After seismic damage from the 1989 Loma Prieta earthquake, the Berkeley Unified School District razed the Environmental Yard and restored its macadam surface; standardized equipment rests on mulch in anther section; a small garden is the only reflection of what had been there before. Parents demanded something "safer" and more predictable, where it would be easier for them to observe their children.

The lesson from our own past is that we should proceed cautiously. We should be on the lookout for the best models to emulate, appreciating that our own history has been fashioned by those who simulate nature or those who effectively construct it. Americans have a different outdoor ethos than most Scandinavians. Even when they have constructed their nature, Scandinavians feel more comfortable in it because they appreciate nature as a way to confront risk. For Scandinavians, but not necessarily for Americans, spending many hours in nature is "looked upon as an important part of growing up and becoming a sensible and well-functioning human being."[14]

Nonetheless, we need to be aware of Scandinavian models, particularly those seen most frequently at Norwegian kindergartens.[15] There, day care facilities might have a "traditional" playground, where kids are outside four or five hours per day, or a naturalized one, where kids spend six or seven hours a day outside. In either instance, the curriculum — self-exploration, play, and learning personal responsibility — meshes with the outdoor environment. The traditional Norwegian playground could have trees or rocks to climb; knives for whittling; and an unprotected pond 150 feet away. There is some fencing; the trees are not very dense. Still, as some commentators have noted, "Children handling knives and saws, climbing high up in trees and cliffs, and sledding at high speed down steep snowy hills are common in most Norwegian child care institutions."[16] Kids find inventive ways to use nature and non-natural materials: "They pile boxes to climb upon, they play-fight a lot, and sometimes they even play-fight on the roof of the playhouse." They also "love to swing, and sometimes they twist the swing so they spin around in high speed. They also jump off the swings in very high speed."

The Norwegian nature playground offers similar experiences, but without fencing or any equipment, just "nature elements such as climbing trees, rock wall/cliffs, grassy hills and fields, and a dense forest."[17] And yet, a recent survey of seventeen hundred Norwegian kindergartens has shown that during 2012, only 10 percent of children received injuries, and 97.9 percent of those needed only "a Band-Aid or some comfort." The remaining injuries, mostly broken bones or concussions, are considered moderate; only 0.2 percent are serious. There are no age differences in injuries, although more boys than girls incur minor injuries. There are no gender differences when it comes to moderate or serious injuries.[18]

Entering Nature

Since American kids no longer regularly play in woods, it is even more surprising that a children's museum might come up with the right blend of architecture and an untapped natural space. A project in New York City combines unadulterated nature, fine architecture, advanced technology, and a meeting place for seniors. Part of the Staten Island Children's Museum and sited on the historic property of Snug Harbor Cultural Center, this inclusive project accommodates several needs and populations. It is a fine example of how forward-thinking architects can work with an enterprising museum director to extend an architectural program. The architects and clients benefited from the fact that this is not officially a play space, which gave them more flexibility; and the museum staff are very lenient in letting kids enthusiastically find their own opportunities.

The Staten Island Children's Museum needed a permanent, covered spot where children could have lunch while on field trips. They also wanted a place to host festivals, at least four times a year. Marpillero Pollak Architects' solution is a dramatic tent that gives an edge to a broad, expansive meadow. It offers shaded public space where kids can bring brown bags and where (after they have eaten and left), seniors can set up their card tables for games of canasta or mah-jongg. The active seniors seem a fitting tribute to the oldest part of the Snug Harbor site, a place that once hosted a nineteenth-century retirement home for seamen. The seamen were housed in a nearby purpose-built complex that is now considered one of the finest examples of American Greek Revival architecture.

This airy, open-sided tent is light, energy responsible, and welcoming.

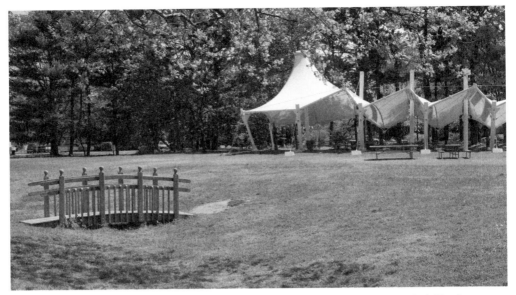

FIGURE 6.1 | *Marpillero Pollak Architects, entrance to Staten Island Children's Museum (2012), New York City. Photograph by Robert S. Solomon, 2013.*

The architects formed translucent fiberglass into a shape that recalls nautical sailcloth. Photovoltaic fabric cells embedded into the tent provide an energy source for strong spotlights that illuminate the site each night. One of the short ends of the tent includes concrete housing for mechanical and electrical backups; a battery-charging station is there for any adult who comes by. Structural masts, which slant like trees, hold up the roof, which slopes, off-center, toward the sun. Each mast of the tent has a drip hole so that water does not accumulate on the surface of the tent. The water trickles into round, flat cisterns that are filled with small rocks. For young children, the rocks are playthings to throw in any direction; helpful maintenance workers return them at the end of each day.

The museum, in addition to having an easy-going attitude toward how kids use the rocks, recognizes the grassy meadow as another play area. This green space, which stretches between the tent structure and the museum entrance, descends gently. Small kids can roll down the hills; older ones get to run all over and experience the topographic changes. During storms, the swails fill with water, giving young visitors a new play area for the few days until the water recedes. Children are also free to investigate the shallow but dense woods that are on the other side of the tent.

On a much larger scale, Carve, the Amsterdam public design firm that conceived of the play street on Potgieterstraat, had an opportunity to create nature play in the revitalization of Meer Park.[19] Meer Park is a large facility on the eastern edge of Amsterdam, outside the historic center. At the time that Carve received the commission, local sports clubs maintained individual spaces along a linear strip. Each club (such as biking, skating, basketball, or fencing) occupied a separately enclosed (and often burglarized) clubhouse. Carve had to find a way to rejuvenate the area, to make it safer and more appealing by providing different opportunities for a variety of age groups and interests beyond sports.

Carve's solution was to organize the site along a central spine that is also a deep, usable entrance. Today the sports clubs exist in the same spots, but they now open up to the central strip of built-up land. This plinth is directional, leading visitors from the parking lot to the new playground at the end. Along the way, pedestrians encounter extra-large picnic tables with barbeque grills. Aligned in a row, these tables provide a respite where families can gather; they also provide a visual clue that leads eyes to the end. Even though the park is open twenty-four hours a day, the number of thefts has decreased because this is a more open environment; there are more visitors with less of the feeling that it is a fortification.

The playground, at the climax of the central spine, easily mixes nature with man-made additions. There are no fences; a meandering stream is

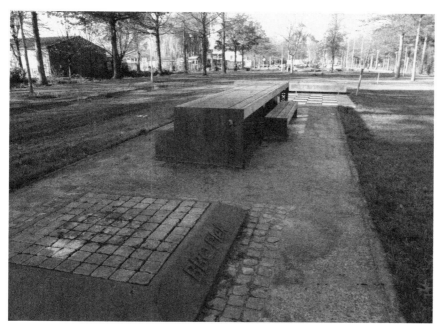

FIGURE 6.2 | *Carve, Meer Park (2010), Amsterdam. The picnic tables form an axis to direct visitors to the playground beyond. Author's photograph, 2013.*

nearby. In addition to the specially designed play structure, the play area includes a bouldering wall. Unlike "play" or imitation walls, this is the real thing, as far as size and difficulty. The material is concrete; even professional boulderers, one of whom helped with the design, can use it for practice. The wall is next to a grassy hill. Since this hill sits over the main gas system of Amsterdam, Carve had to make sure that it was extremely light, yet strong enough to hold an embedded sliding structure with high crossed tube slides.

Nearby, the stream meanders near the play structure. It soon becomes clear that the far bank of the stream could be for play, too. An unprotected clatter bridge joins the two sides. The Dutch take a light-hearted approach toward having their waterways, including this stream, without fencing. They are not being cavalier but are displaying their deep-seated belief that parents have to make sure their offspring have basic survival skills. Every parent responsibly sees to it that his four-year-old learns to swim and his child knows what to do if he ends up in water with his clothes on. Liberated from worrying about drownings, Carve was able to provide paths along the

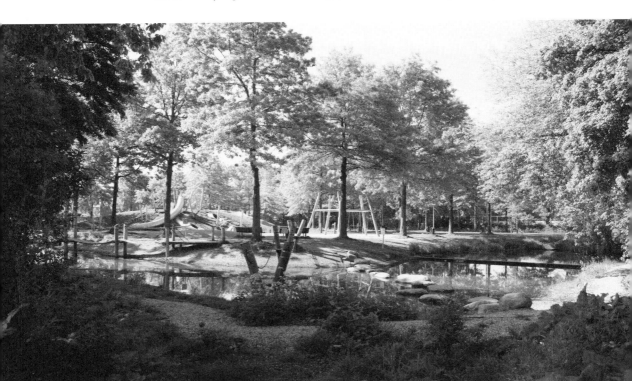

FIGURE 6.3 | *Carve, Meer Park (2010), Amsterdam. There are areas for play on both banks of the stream. Courtesy of Carve.nl. (Plate 7)*

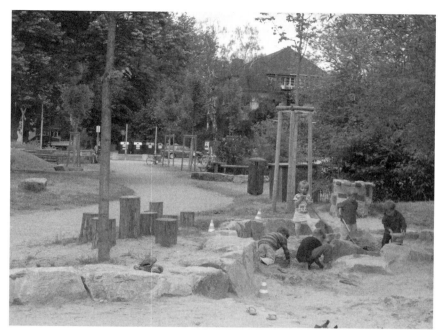

FIGURE 6.4 | *Vauban (Freiburg), Germany, play area.*
Copyright Tim Gill (www.rethinkingchildhood.com).

stream as well as a stack of logs with a simple tunnel through it, right alongside the water.

Nature on Several Scales

Nature playgrounds fit well with the planning principles of greening
our cities. Freiburg, Germany, which was built anew after the bombings of
World War II, illustrates the comfortable fit between green planning and
nature play.[20] One of Germany's greenest cities (both politically and ecologically) and situated very close to the natural wonders of the Black Forest,
Freiburg has been especially welcoming to efforts to encourage a walking
and biking culture by improving public transportation.

This is especially true in Vauban, a transit-oriented development (TOD)
built on an abandoned 1930s military base within Freiburg. Seventy percent
of residents do not own vehicles. Playgrounds have augmented this healthful and forward-thinking lifestyle. Rather than being overly engineered,
play spaces have sprung up as simple nodes. Playgrounds are especially
plentiful within the interior courtyard of housing units. They supersede
the street, even though the streets have limited traffic.[21] For the youngest
children, this semisheltered space keeps them within a close range of their

homes. They often play on dead trees that have been stripped of bark and placed on sand or pea gravel. Parents are nearby; kids can reach their houses quickly if they need them, but young children can also be left pretty much on their own.

When kids play with nature, here, it seems like an ordinary development; it is an extension of the way the community developed. It never feels as if these play areas have been imposed, because they mesh with the landscape as well as with their community values of low energy consumption, walking, and retention of nature. There are sandpits and rock outcroppings along many of the interior paths, and some of these play spaces do come close to the street. Some of the areas take advantage of the setting; others arrange the rocks, tree stubs, and sand. In summer, kids get to play in deep ravines with high grass along shallow streams; they play in the same place, on ice, in winter. These are usually the sites where rain water runs off and is recycled.

In Denmark, Helle Nebelong, the landscape architect who designed the natural play area in Valby Park, has dedicated herself to working within the framework of natural playgrounds. When she says that nature provides a way so that "children have to use their full bodies and minds to explore and manage their surroundings,"[22] her words seem to echo scientist Adele Diamond, who declared that the best way to learn, especially for young children, is to be actively engaged in a task. "Active learning," Nebelong writes, "involves the whole body, all the senses."[23]

Nebelong employed her philosophy at the Murergaarden School in Copenhagen, where it blends well with the Scandinavian approach to extended socialization for young kids. She designed and completed the project in 1998. The site, having been the subject of architectural and design articles and many written treatises on nature play, has become an icon for natural playgrounds.[24] Nebelong teased many natural wonders from this very confined urban space in the gentrifying, but still often poor, area of Norboro.

This site posed a design challenge because it needed to provide play opportunities for children ranging in age from birth to fourteen. Nebelong's job was to unify the space (which is open twenty-four hours a day and is available to neighbors at all nonschool hours) and to make it interesting enough to appeal to children throughout the large age spread. The existing playground included two separate levels—a six-foot elevation change—occupied by separate age groups (zero to six and seven to fourteen) and separated by a fence. In addition to the students' needs, Nebelong also had to consider the wishes of a large group that was active in the planning pro-

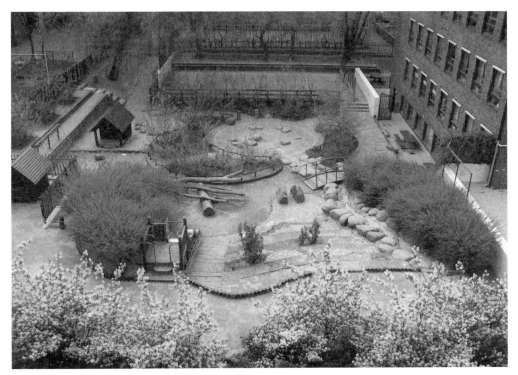

FIGURE 6.5 | *Helle Nebelong, Murergaarden School yard (1998), Copenhagen, Denmark. Nebelong took this photo in 2005. Courtesy of Helle Nebelong.*

cess, including teachers and administrators of this and other nearby day care centers. Their requests included varied surfaces, water play, and hiding spots.

Nebelong fulfilled many of their desires: varied stones connect the upper and lower levels, thereby supplying changes in terrain and texture. Other stones and tree stumps outline a paddling pool at the bottom level. In the summer, teachers use a hose to wet the rock terraces and to fill the pool. A few small bridges pass over culverts. An old tree trunk in a sand area on the bottom level provides a climbing obstacle for small fry and a welcome place for older children to hang out. Deep bushes, perfect for hiding and exploring, appear throughout the site; the flowers are seasonal and therefore attract insects and butterflies. Willow trees, placed near the paddling pool, provide stems for art projects. If need be, a small area can be cordoned off for nursery-age kids. All of this was accomplished for a total cost of 750,000 Danish krone (approximately $130,000 at the time).

Two new environmental education centers in Northern Europe show how the idea of nature often is most convincing when it is on a grand scale.

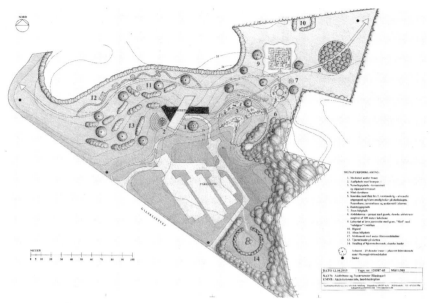

FIGURE 6.6 | *Helle Nebelong, plan of Hindsgavl Deer Park at Middelfart on Funen Island (2013), Denmark. Tim Ebikon hand-colored the drawing. Courtesy of Helle Nebelong.*

Once again, Helle Nebelong's skills have been put to good use in establishing a place where children can interact with nature. The site is the Hindsgavl Deer Park of Middelfart on Funen Island in Denmark. The municipality had already built an Activity and Outdoor Centre (AART Architects, 2012) within a 170-acre wildlife park. The town asked Nebelong to take charge of the landscape, including specific play areas for children. Her site descends down a steep hill and almost surrounds the activity center. Nebelong, keeping the site as undisturbed as possible, has used winding gravel paths to guide the travel of adults and children.

From a child's perspective, the key feature of the garden is its collection of mazes of different sizes and types. Thirteen mazes made from plantings, rocks, or logs invite kids to run, jump, and test their swinging skills within the comfortable reassurance of natural surroundings. Nebelong also dug an amphitheater into a hill so that there can be outdoor demonstrations for kids. Collectively, these features assure children that they can be inventive and create their own play activities using only the natural surroundings.

The Environment Education Center (De Drijfsijs) in Amsterdam, which opened in 2012, shows that free access and lush beauty can give an environmental commission a separate life of its own. Carve has created a magical

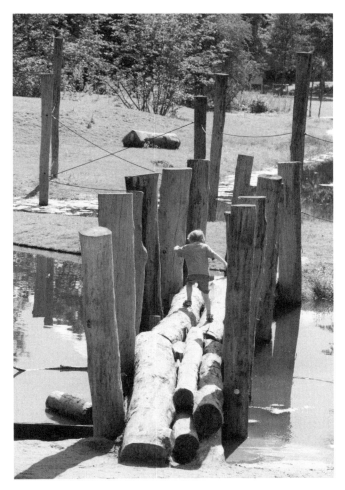

FIGURE 6.7
Carve. Environmental Education Center at Sloterpark (2012), Amsterdam, Netherlands. Courtesy of Carve.nl.

space for kids either to learn about nature with guides from the Education Center, or just to come and experience on their own. Carve worked with the NiewWest district of the city for this facility, maintained in the city's largest park, Sloterpark.

Participation is what sets this facility apart from a picturesque park. Adjacent to a school, the property can be used by anyone at any time. There are neither barriers nor fencing. Carve has devised a variety of strategies that will draw kids in. Alternatively, kids can go off and invent, dig, or construct anything they choose, in swamp or brush. The designers carefully piled wood twigs in hope that children will climb on them and also discover the creatures that nest there. The water, filled with logs, is appealing and attractive to kids. Some of the logs, placed at angles, are challenging for climbing. Others, laid out as a tree trunk path, offer kids a more direct way to cross

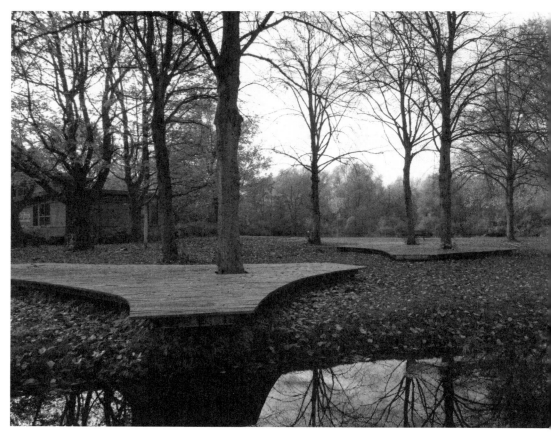

FIGURE 6.8 | *Carve. Environmental Education Center at Sloterpark (2012), Amsterdam, Netherlands. The designers envision parents relaxing and reading on these handsome benches while the offspring explore the rest of the park. Author's photograph, 2012.*

the water. An overhead zip line is irresistible for children who want a more daring way to hang over the wet landscape. Another area of water has a bridge; there is a rail on one side so that wheelchairs can come close to the edge. All water is recycled, and the hills were built from dirt excavated on site so that no new dirt had to be brought in. Elger Blitz, of Carve, insisted that elegant free-form wooden benches be placed around trees. These are in one area of the park, close to the entrance. Blitz envisioned parents hanging out, reading, or chatting, while the kids immersed themselves in nature.

Uprooting Nature: Animals, Trees

Nature has to include animals, something Carve tried to promote in the woodpile at the environment center. While more and more school-yards in the United States are introducing gardening or outdoor nature classrooms, there is less attention to using animals as part of a schoolyard experience. At Svartlamon Kindergarten (the "art and culture school") in Trondheim, animals are part of the everyday schoolyard experience.

Before working on the kindergarten, architects Geir Brendeland and Olav Kristoffersen (Brendeland & Kristoffersen, Trondheim) had previously won recognition for their design of a low-cost halfway house in the neighborhood. They used untreated wood in pursuit of fine design. After the housing was completed, a nearby car dealer attempted to sell his building and its land to a developer. The neighbors, part of the alternative Svartlamon district, protested that what the community needed was a proper kindergarten: up until then, childcare had been a cooperative venture, with the parents taking turns watching children.

Brendeland & Kristoffersen's transformed the former dealership into a private kindergarten, one that emphasizes the arts and follows the tenets of the Reggio-Emilia network of schools. As they had in the halfway house, the architects used raw wood so that kids can hang their art projects or paint directly on the walls. Kids can see the outdoors clearly from the front-facing classrooms. A wooden wall, made to look like concrete, encloses the space where children play. The barrier is necessary because the abutting road has heavy truck traffic. Driftwood and climbing apparatuses make up the official play equipment. The ubiquitous hill, found in kindergarten play spaces, is also at the side. The real draw is a space for animals that adjoins the play area. Kids enjoy visiting the sheep who reside there; they see them being shorn and find out how wool is spun. They are also tremendously excited each spring when the lambs arrive. The notable aspect is that the sheep are an integral part of the routine each day; the animals are not really pets or even farm animals for the young students, because they enjoy them as part of the natural environment. The school has adapted nature so that it is "ordinary" in the best possible way.[25]

The playground takes advantage of the ReMida recycling center adjoining where the sheep are housed. Following Reggio-Emilia principles, the center (part of an international network of similar facilities) provides usable waste for art and construction projects. All the schools in the city may take advantage of the offerings. For the children at the Svartlamon kindergarten it takes on distinct meaning because it is a source of materials they can use — on the spot — for self-initiated building projects. Migrating between the sheep and the recycling spaces, the children combine the open-ended activities of an adventure playground with the daily rituals that real animals perform. They balance their time with manmade materials and a more natural setting.

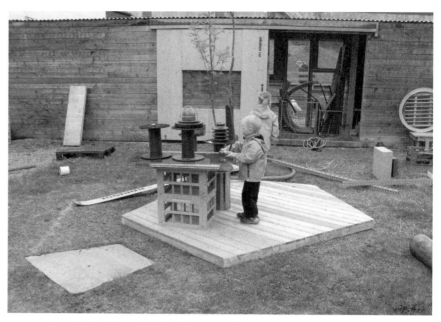

FIGURE 6.9 | *Brendeland & Kristoffersen, outdoor space at Svartlamon Kindergarten (2007), Trondheim, Norway. The view is from the recycling center (next door) with a view toward the sheep that stay at the school and the playground hill, beyond. Courtesy of Pål Bøyesen and ReMida, Trondheim. (Plate 8)*

Ideally, nature play is messy and malleable. There should be endless twigs, rocks, and sand to manipulate. We should not forget that more refined nature, effectively "uprooted nature," can play a role too. It is sustainable. It can be fanciful and useful. Michael van Valkenburgh Associates (MVVA) did something interesting in their plan for North Grant Park in Chicago. Located east of Millennium Park, the area will be named Maggie Daley Park in memory of the wife of former mayor Richard Daley. Like Millennium Park, Daley Park sits over an underground parking garage. When the garage roof needed repair, it spurred the need to remove the old park and build a newer version. MVVA has designed an Enchanted Forest for younger kids as one of the highlights.[26] Since trees from this old site could not be replanted, MVVA stripped them and positioned them upside down. They provide a sudden surprise, filled with whimsy, for children coming into one section of the new park.

Patrick Dougherty builds on the sense of enchantment in his artwork, most of which has found homes at universities or in art museums (for example, the garden at Dumbarton Oaks in Washington, DC; Middlebury College in Vermont; or the Contemporary Art Museum in Honolulu). Trained as an art historian and sculptor, Dougherty switched more than thirty years ago from more traditional sculpture materials to environmental art composed of saplings. He elects to do only ten or twelve projects per year. For the Bay Area Discovery Museum at Fort Baker in Sausalito, CA, he created a multichamber piece where kids could be awed by the stick structure, hide in small rooms, or even jab at the willow twigs. His piece lasted seven years because the museum was diligent in its maintenance; the normal lifespan for this "living art" is two years.[27]

Within the museum's outdoor "Lookout Cove" play area, Peekaboo Palace (2012) has replaced Dougherty's first effort, which did eventually wear out; the site is the same but Dougherty expanded his piece to include more rooms. Peekaboo Palace is set back, not immediately visible from a well-thought-out area with boat paraphernalia and a working gravel construction site. Kids have to roam a bit to find it. When they come to it, it is not immediately visible if there is a main entrance. There are several paths. Once inside, they can explore several different nooks and experience varied light sources. They can climb in and out of the windows, but the undulating roof is made purposefully to discourage them from tackling that. Kids

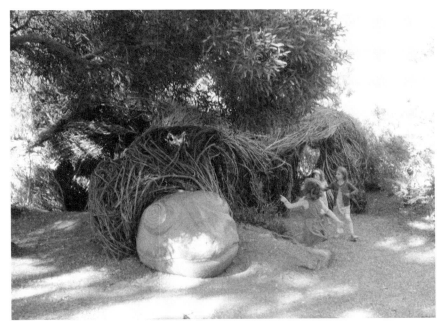

FIGURE 6.10 | *Patrick Dougherty, Peekaboo Palace (2012), installation at Bay Area Discovery Museum, Sausalito, California. Dougherty matches his installations to the site. He works at the site during the entire construction and hand selects volunteers for the building process. Author's photograph, 2013.*

quickly learn that there is no set route; the intricacy of the willows is engaging in its own right. They are surprised when they find a granite sculpture of a frog head (Marcia Donahue), one that was already on the site and that Dougherty incorporated into his composition.

The final cost for the new piece was in the range of slightly less than $40,000. At first glance that seems like a steep price for a temporary structure. In fact, it is possible to argue that it is cost effective. The piece is unique, so the kids' experiences cannot be replicated. This museum is conscientious to make the stick sculpture last six or seven years; off-the-shelf equipment, by comparison, can cost as much or more without offering any intrigue, and it is often disposed of almost as quickly.

"Uprooted nature" can also be powerfully evocative and enticingly playable. HHA (the same firm that designed Geopark) devised an unusual piece for a Victoria & Albert Museum exhibition (2010): "Architects Build Small Spaces." Asked to provide something whimsical, the architects thought about trees. Trees had supplied lively childhood experiences for their own young years, when they played in the forest; there was no artificial distinction between "play space" and where they chose to play. The architects, who wanted to make the connection that children who play in the forest also navigate between the uplifting and the mundane, called their piece Ratatosk. The name refers to the mythical squirrel (literally "drill tooth") who gnawed at trees and who passed messages to the Norse gods. By participating in the life of the Norse gods and the continuing life cycle of the tree, Ratatosk positioned himself as a player in the flux of the eternal and ordinary worlds. HHA used every part of five trees so that these become a single climbing piece that reinvents and recombines the old tree by giving it a "new life."[28] HHA chose an ash tree for their project; it is strong and grows quickly, so its sustainability quotient is excellent. They split the trees vertically, then digitally prepared them for milling. The interiors are therefore smooth. A ring on the ground holds them together. The exterior bark, stripped from the tree was placed in a pillow for climbing that sits on the floor of the sculpture. The branches were thinly sliced and linked to create a canopy.

The V&A commission has led to the possibility that there might be a forest of Ratatosks in the future. The concept has already played a part at Skadbergbakken, a new residential development that is being constructed outside of Stavanger. HHA did the master plan for this new community (single-family homes, small apartment blocks, units for the elderly), which will be adjacent to a new train line. They added three dead trees, connected by rope for climbing, in an area where the preschoolers play.

The concept of using nature is a powerful one. We should take advantage of it—in both its living and dead states—when it is appropriate. We need to be especially vigilant in evaluating it because it is currently such a hot—and not necessarily stringently assessed—topic. Too often, we follow it too blindly or, conversely, discard it. After Super Storm Sandy (October 2012), in which old, healthy trees were uprooted in America's Northeast (New York City, alone, may have lost more than ten thousand), only a few agencies thought of stripping fallen trees of their bark and employing them as climbing structures. The Prospect Park Alliance in Brooklyn used those, as well as trees lost earlier during hurricane Irene and some that were felled during a 2010 tornado; these became the underpinning of the Donald & Barbara Zucker Natural Exploration Area, which takes advantage—in the best way—of nature's whims.

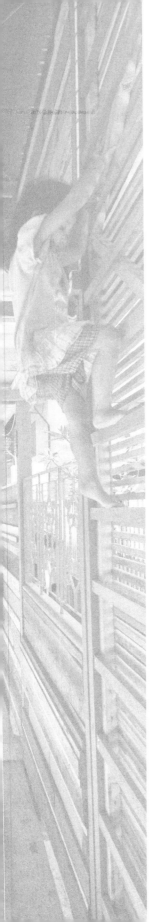

7 Paths

NOW WE NEED TO CONFIDENTLY PURSUE new paths and policies in order to create vibrant areas equal to or even better than the ones we have already viewed. Let's think less about "playground" and more about a generalized "playscape" or even "play site," spaces that merge with their surroundings and are part of a broader context. We have to value (and include) architects and landscape architects in how we proceed; and we have to find solutions that are cost effective and sustainable. We need to tap into children's real, often shrouded, desires. If we don't adopt these changes, most American playground sites will remain banal; kids will continue to be ghettoized; use will continue to drop; and funding will dry up. We will have lost a chance not only to rethink play sites but also to enrich our environment and broaden our individual lives.

Containment

Containment is no longer a viable solution. We need to break down barriers that are physical and perceptual. If we begin to switch our frame of reference from enclosed playgrounds to more open play sites, we soon see how outdated and restrictive the existing equipment and high fences are. The objective is to develop intergenerational space, with an emphasis on children and places to play, in order to help kids become mature, independent young adults. We cannot do that if play sties are exclusionary. Adults have to weigh their fears and realize that their angst about strangers may be a result of what they have heard, not a factor of what is true. Instead of considering how to keep people out, we should think of how to draw them in. Aase Eriksen argued in favor of playscapes as opposed to playgrounds in 1985; we should, finally, be acting on her recommendations. Even earlier, in the late 1960s, many architects, planners, and other advocates for better public spaces were demanding webs of small, unfenced, open areas. These are not new ideas; we need to rethink readapt, and readopt them.[1]

Architects, Landscape Architects, Artists

The examples in the previous chapters show how artists—sculptors as well as architects and landscape architects—have the ability to be imaginative, sensitive to needs, and aware of a sense of place. In several instances, such as Helen & Hard's work or Superuse Studios designs, the materials are abundant and inexpensive. The general public thinks that employing artists will increase the price when, in fact, they may lower it because they are not hemmed in by having to use conventional playground equipment. Similarly, artwork not designated as a playground is often exempt from adhering to America's safety guidelines.

Percent for Art programs, so far thwarted in the United States when it comes to play areas, could be key. Site specific and unique, these have the best chance of evoking memories and creating the realm of place. These could sponsor artwork that enhances children's outdoor experiences and helps to defray costs in the same way they do in Trondheim. The creation of these programs in American municipalities since 1959 dovetailed with the creation of some of the wonderfully inventive playgrounds that architects and landscape architects devised in the 1960s. Yet, in Philadelphia, the site of the first American Percent for Art Program, the ending was not a happy one. The city turned down a request to fund a playground designed by sculptor and playground designer Joe Brown. The city proclaimed that a playground could not be sculpture. Philadelphia's severe pronouncement, followed by later federal guidelines, discouraged many American artists from entering the playground design arena. With forceful encouragement, both city administrators and artists might now be ready to reconsider.

Designers and Kids

Artists may have been absent from designs for play, but children have not been ignored in recent decades, especially when it comes to selecting equipment from a catalog. Well-meaning programs, calculated to incorporate the designs of children into playground design, have pushed kids into the design phase (often with great fanfare and public attention) but have often failed in their mission. Once we say that the design is being turned over to kids—something that happens daily in America—we are usually asking them to think of post and deck and other off-the-shelf equipment. The idea that children, left to their own devices, can design a play area is silly and sentimental; it also maintains the status quo and thwarts innovation. The urge to have children take charge of playground design may reflect how difficult it often is to gain support for a play project. Turn the design over to kids, and it cynically becomes a winning notion. Dollars pour in. Bringing in children may also be a misinterpretation of the 1990 UN Convention on the Rights of the Child, which says that children should be able to express opinions on actions that affect them; they also have the right to play and to recreation.

Designers should certainly listen to young clients, learn from them, interpret what they long for, and create the places that kids don't even know they desire. Kids' drawings could play a part if these reflect their daily lives, or even fantasies. In several instances, parks incorporate the drawings into permanent mosaics or murals that grace the new playground and aid the feeling of stewardship among young users. In the United States, the Trust for Public Land (TPL) has led the way in marshaling the enthusiasm of young people into permanent displays. As part of their Parks for People division and their commitment to "creative place making," they have often brought artists into the design process. For Bella Vista playground in Oakland, CA, TPL commissioned metalsmith Eric Powell to design an entrance gate; Powell incorporated found objects, many unearthed by children at home or on the old playground site, into the final design. At other sites, TPL artists have worked with high school students who did the actual fabrication of glass and ceramic tiles that were placed on playgrounds.[2]

Roger Hart, the codirector of the Children's Environments Research Group at the City University of New York, points out the limitations of asking kids to design a playground. Children are imaginative, but they can draw only what they have seen. Asking kids to "design" a playground will therefore keep the status quo.[3] Instead, Hart suggests asking kids questions that will illuminate their basic fears, hopes, and desires. The questions are almost always indirect. He queries them about what they like to do, what's scary, what they're not supposed to do, and what makes them feel comfortable. His strategy also involves intense observation of how children play and interact.

The cooperative Norwegian architectural firm TYIN Tegnestue Architects (Yashar Hanstad and Andreas Gjetsen are the founding principals) has devised its own strategies to elicit kids' point of view in projects for underserved communities in Southeast Asia.[4] Their approach meshes well with their call for an "Architecture of Necessity" (a term that has been around for about a decade) and "social sustainability," a term they coined.[5] This award-winning firm (the winners of the European Prize for Architecture and the City 2.0 Prize, both in 2012) along with students, many of whom come from the Norwegian University of Science and Technology, has learned how to get young people to tell their own stories. When they ask children to draw, the purpose is to let the kids draw what they know, not what they want.

For the Klong Toey area of Bangkok, TYIN devised a combination playground, sports space, and community center on a lot that had at one time been a soccer field but subsequently had been an abandoned site (approximately 15 x 38 feet) where garbage accumulated. The facility is located in a tough slum where 140,000 people live in substandard, unsanctioned housing. Violence and drugs are rampant. The architects talk about establishing a quiet area for talking and playing that can provide a refuge from the dangers of living in this place and that could possibly become a magnet for additional social services. They hoped that the residents would aspire to more local control and activism once they saw what could be achieved. They saw this space—like any good playground—as a site of continual change and improvement.

TYIN asked five- to ten-year-old kids about their home life: What's it like, and what do they do there? The Norwegians noticed, for instance, that children always included an intense sunlight in the drawings of their home life. It soon became apparent that shade was a luxury for these children and should be a major goal of the design. They also asked kids to bring in something that was not needed from home and about which they would want to talk. One child brought in some glass. The designers then thought about the object's possible uses and purpose. It became the genesis of hanging lights that keep the site well lighted at night.

The result, which took a year to plan and three weeks to construct, is the Klong Toey Community Lantern. The title "Lantern" is appropriate and another reference to "glass," because the building is meant to be secure and protecting in the same way that a lantern shields light. It is inspiring to see how much was done here. The drawings the children made, which showed them looking down at their peers playing below, were a source of inspiration for the designers to implement a two-story (on two sides), fifteen-foot-high ensemble. Using old timber and metal as well as new building materials, the architects created an oblong building with a central courtyard. They salvaged local metal for the mezzanine. There is a stage for performances and meetings. Casting a concrete base was a triumph over obstacles, especially during the rainy season.

The wood is layered to present a permeable side to the street and a more enclosed face inside. A walkway/seating area runs between these two "walls." The courtyard, with a basketball net at one end, is also the soccer pitch. Its narrow ends are semiclosed to the street. Kids can sit on either level to watch the sports action; on the first level they can sit on swings. They love to climb to different heights along the wood walls, exactly as the designers

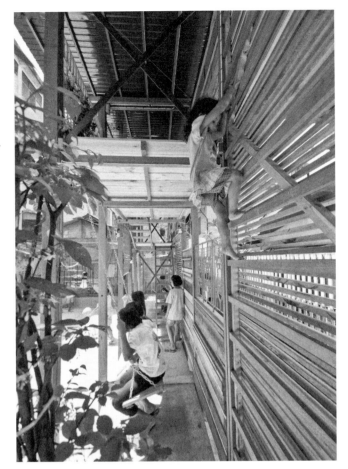

FIGURE 7.1

TYIN Tegnestue Architects, Klong Toey Community Lantern (2011), Bangkok, Thailand. Photo by Pasi Aalto. Courtesy of TYIN Tegnestue Architects. (Plate 9)

intended. TYIN principal Yashar Hanstad says that there are stairs, but the children find every opportunity not to use them. That is exactly what the designers had hoped.

The Future of Public Venues

We have arrived at a time when both playgrounds and libraries are in danger of becoming irrelevant. These institutions have parallel histories; both are in crisis today. The public library appeared first, in the mid-nineteenth century; public playgrounds began popping up before the next century, although their focus and purpose were originally different from what developed later. Each of these originally urban institutions extended services to throngs of immigrants; each intended to improve lives. Each is deeply rooted in our collective past and each is affected today by technology, changing patterns of use and need, and varied types of patrons. Libraries, to their credit, are making vigorous assessments of how to be useful to average citizens. A few have reconceptualized their form and function.[6]

Other building types that previously had not imagined roles as public squares are taking up the challenge of reinvention. The Oslo Opera House might be one of the best examples (Snøhetta). Broad exterior ramps on the sides of the building extend from a wide plaza to the top where they join another wide promenade at the back of the building. None of these enhancements are necessary for opera or ballet. They exist because the architects wanted to redefine the "town square" by providing a space to stroll any time of day or night. Similarly, the Casa da Musica (OMA, 2005) in Porto, Portugal, has a broad plaza of undulating planes, arranged expressly so skateboarders may infuse life into a once neglected part of the city. This music hall's educators are also working with skateboarders to incorporate their sounds into musical compositions.[7] Surely, play sites that are meant to be large public venues could be similarly innovative. We should be thinking in terms of spaces that, like a good library or music hall, expand daily experience. Playgrounds need to undergo a similar transformation if they are to remain indispensable to a community.

At the same time, we have to resist acting—out of frustration—independently. We should be wary of privatization filling the void if public spaces no longer draw children. We will see more and more pay-per-day indoor amusement centers with generic environments; kids have no personal connections either to the place itself or to the other children playing there. Alternatively, we may see desperate parents taking actions that inadvertently undermine support for public projects. Blogger and former Internet entrepreneur Mike Lanza is a good example. He has transformed the front and rear yards of his home in Menlo Park, California, into Playborhood.[8] Lanza, who wanted to guarantee that his own children would have plenty of time outdoors and abundant opportunities to hang out with their neighbors, feels passionately about his kids' development and their need for interesting outdoor experiences. He has taken it upon himself to provide water features and homemade climbing/resting stations in his front yard and to make this available to neighborhood kids. While we can marvel at his dedication and generosity, we should not ignore the fact that he has effectively co-opted public space by turning his previously private realm into a public venture. He has used his own time, money, and land to create something that simulates public space. Perhaps unwittingly, he is acknowledging that he has to provide scintillating experiences that no longer exist in a local nearby park.

Reconceptualizing Risk: Toward a National Policy

Three types of fear prevent us from building and sustaining rich play sites for kids. We have parents who are genuinely fearful about their children's safety. Somewhat allied to that fear, we have parents who don't believe that their offspring are capable of making good choices or protecting themselves. We also have an unfounded fear of strangers, especially when they arrive without children in a public space. While some of these phobias are so ingrained that they could be considered markers of our culture, it is possible to alter, or at least shift, some of them so that they will be less debilitating for all of us. We need to let parents know that they are not aiding their kids when they are overprotective, unsupportive, and fearful of strangers. We have to counter fear with the belief that kids can watch out for themselves.

Years ago, the playground was the first place where kids could separate from their parents—the place where kids could learn to be independent. With so many fearful parents in our midst, we have to turn this idea on its head. Let's teach parents how essential independence is for children, and let's urge parents to look at any play site as their first place to grant self-sufficiency to their kids. Play spaces should be the parents' lab, the place where they can take their "first steps" in letting their children accept responsibility for their own actions. It's the place where, for a short time, they can put their own fears on hold.

Sometimes, adults—even teachers—have to put their own fears aside. Small actions by designers can help American adults to stop hovering: for instance, providing seating that is relatively far enough away from playground equipment sends a message that children should be playing on their own. It is possible to build a playscape so that it provides the necessary environment for adults to relax and watch from a distance. Mathew Urbanski, who is principal in Michael van Valkenburgh Associates (MVVA), understands this well. Urbanski and his team—as the landscape designers who have just begun to plan a massive park in Tulsa, Oklahoma, that the local George Kaiser Family Foundation is supporting—have included a high and sizable seating area for adults. He describes it as a "panopticon" pyramid where adults will be able to sit and relax yet also keep a distant eye on young folks. Urbanski sees this as necessary for kids and their freedom; he also sees it as compulsory to the success of the park. He believes that the comfort of parents has a direct impact on how long kids stay. If parents do not find satisfying places to spend time, they will likely pack up their children and go somewhere else.[9]

In addition to altering personal perceptions and attitudes toward risk, we need high-level institutional change. Up until now, adjustments such as state recreational immunity laws have been sporadic; several states have enacted this type of legislation, which exempts local public spaces (usually including playgrounds and skate parks) from being suited unless there has been gross negligence. There have been unintended consequences, in that municipalities have deferred maintenance when they thought the immunity law would prevent them from being sued.[10] The immunity laws, once seen as a great hope, now appear to be a possible dead end. Perhaps there will be a way to counteract their ineffectiveness with a different type of future legislation.

Right now, we need intrepid actions. We have to question federal guidelines that further "surplus safety," which obscures "the benefits associated with exciting, challenging, and stimulating play."[11] Institutions in the United Kingdom have pursued a more thoughtful, liberating approach that embraces risk-benefit analysis over a zero-risk policy. In the 1970s and 1980s, the British, too, saw children as needing protection, and they continued to highlight worst-case possibilities as to what could harm kids.[12] While individual parents may still subscribe to that philosophy, their government's outlook has changed in impressive ways.

The British have made huge advances in altering that atmosphere, and they are showing that systemic change is possible when there is strong leadership and smart advocacy. The national environment altered in the late 1990s, perhaps reflecting the emergence of "New Labour" (Tony Blair became prime minister in 1997), with its broad social policy, emphasis on personal responsibility, and public-private partnerships. On a national level, the Play Safety Forum (PSF) began to take a stand against excessive safety and to argue for a more balanced approach. The composition of the PSF was remarkable: it brought together national leaders of diverse interest groups, including the Royal Society of the Prevention of Accidents (RoSPA); the Children Play Council (which became Play England and is managed by the National Children's Bureau); representatives of play organizations from Wales, Scotland, and Northern Ireland; the National Playing Fields Association (which subsequently became Fields in Trust); and manufacturers of play equipment.

PSF issued their first significant paper in 2002. Entitled "Managing Risk in Play Provision," this document became the framework for a system of assessment keyed to "risk-benefit analysis." The most telling word in the title is "Managing"; this was not a crusade to eliminate or obliterate risk.

Between 2002 and 2012 the PSF issued a series of refinements; simultaneously, local play areas received a huge infusion of money from the National Lottery. By 2008, the federal funding for play totaled £390 million (about $600 million). A British government document published that fall announced a "ten-year Children's Plan that aims to make England the best place in the world to grow up."[13]

In that same year, 2008, Play England produced an implementation guide (Tim Gill, Bernard Spiegal, and David Ball were the authors) that codified how risk-benefit analysis works. It's an intriguing system because it does not involve scoring or any specific "don'ts." Instead, it sets out steps to evaluate each play project: identify the benefit; identify the risk; compare the options (for example, is there something that has to be eliminated? Is there something that is too tame and not challenging?); research precedents and locate comparisons; make a judgment and follow through with implementation. As Tim Gill, has said, the process asks people to evaluate play spaces on the basis of common sense and whether having a particular object or piece of equipment is reasonable. An official government document ("Staying Safe, the Government's Safeguarding Strategy"), published in 2008, sounded a similar line on risk by recognizing that "'wrapping children in cotton wool,' or minimizing all risks, however small, for fear of litigation, was having a negative impact on children's play opportunities and their more general freedom to explore and encounter the world, appropriate to their age."[14]

Most significantly, the English Health and Safety Executive (which in the United States would be akin to an amalgam of the Department of Health and Human Services and the Consumer Product Safety Commission) issued its own high-level statement in 2012 (during the coalition government led by Conservative David Cameron and during the same year that the updated manual on Managing Risk in Play Provision Implementation Guide appeared.). This policy statement makes clear that, since we cannot have a world without risk, risk-benefit analysis is a suitable means for implementing play environments. This pronouncement is a crucial key in that it indicates that the highest levels of English government endorse risk-benefit analysis, what Tim Gill refers to as "beneficial risk."[15] The Royal Society of Prevention of Accidents now has a motto: "As safe as necessary, not as safe as possible." That is quite a mantra for RoSPA, "the largest play safety organization in the world."[16] Even the United Nations, which endorsed the Convention on the Rights of the Child, is adapting an approach that asks, "What is safe enough?"[17]

There is already evidence from Britain that their policy is producing

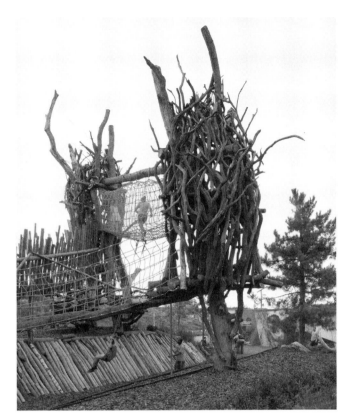

FIGURE 7.2
*erect architecture (playstructure)
and LUC (design landscaping)
(2013), Queen Elizabeth Olympic
Park north playground, London.
This project won the competition
that the London Legacy
Development Corporation
sponsored for one of the sites
left following the 2012 Olympic
Games. Photograph by David
Grandorge. Courtesy of erect
architecture. (Plate 10)*

stunning results. Here are two examples that indicate small and large shifts in attitude. First, the Children's Scrapstore, a program that brings shipping containers (PlayPods) of clean waste products (fabrics, cardboard tubes, computer keyboards) to school yards, is expanding its program. Second, Barbara Kaucky, principal with Susanne Tutsch in the English firm erect architecture, says that the national policy of beneficial risk has liberated their design concepts and has created better clients, ones who can now think more daringly about spaces for children.[18] Their design for the Queen Elizabeth playground is a case in point. The first public section to open (2013) on the former 2012 Olympic site, the playground won the international competition for a play-worthy site based on nature. Erect's solution—which also includes a field house—is a series of carefully orchestrated experiences of water, sand, rope structures, and felled trees. The architects sought to create a way for children to "test limits of courage and ability." The climax is called Scots Pine. To get to these hollowed trees that have been changed into intricate weavings of tree branches, kids have to go across shaky bridges; they can climb up an embankment sheathed by logs; a swing is suspended from the tall tree. It looks tenuous and welcomes kids to find out whether it will be able to support them. Kids (starting at about five years old but now attracting many teens) can make many choices, and it is never totally clear what they will be able to master or overcome. Once other parts of the Olympic site have been reconstructed, this playground will be linked to an existing neighborhood for which it will likely offer an enticing center.

American Actions

The American legal system, admittedly, is rather different from the British. The scheme in the United Kingdom is weighted against bringing lawsuits because the losing plaintiff must pay all legal fees. There is no jury system, which could also be a deterrent to bringing frivolous suits. Three judges, who are presumably well versed in what they are asked to consider, make a determination. The British, who have a long-standing National Health System, also have an educational philosophy that departs in significant ways from ours. Their Early Years Foundation Stage (EYFS), which began in September 2008, is a comprehensive program that emphasizes "safety, health, achievement, making a contribution, and being economically sustainable."[19] The curriculum for children under five encourages risk taking, to the point that one advocate notes that "the challenge for practitioners may be to review the [outdoor] space and to think about ways to increase the risks, rather than minimize them."[20]

Despite these differences, we should nevertheless look across the Atlantic for guidance. If we are going to change the play debate and play sites, we need courageous leadership at the national level that will redefine our acceptance of risk. Following the British lead, we need high-level coalitions, which bring together diverse groups that advocate not just for play but also for urban design, architecture, and park preservation. Physicians, parks departments, manufacturers, and even trial lawyers have to be part of the solution. It is likely that a governmental infrastructure already exists. We already have a CPSC; now we need its leaders to reconsider its mandate and to forge new alliances so that we can inaugurate policies that make sense in the same way as those of our British cousins.

There are already some promising ideas and policies flowing from the ground up (both literally and figuratively), and indications that mayors and local advocates also could be influential in future change. In Washington, DC, OLIN landscape architects are doing the initial studies for Franklin Park. They are considering "a place of 24/7 social engagement"; they are listening to neighbors' suggestions that there be a play space, possibly one without "fenced climbing equipment."[21] The city of Cambridge, Massachusetts, created a report titled "Healthy Parks and Playgrounds" (2009) that acknowledges that play is "experimental, challenging, and sometimes risky."

In Chicago, Mayor Rahm Emanuel made news about playgrounds in 2013. On behalf of the Chicago Park District, the mayor signaled that Chicago would refurbish three hundred playgrounds over five years. The goal was not just to spruce up aging equipment but to be socially and economically responsive. Emanuel wants playgrounds, located within a ten-minute walk of every child's home, to be "a catalyst for a better quality of life and higher standard of living for every Chicagoan."[22] With limited finances, he identified playgrounds as a quick way of getting "the most possible bang for the buck."[23] The park district, which is counting on "specialized mulch" (they have since decided on "engineered wood fiber") as their new ground cover of choice, hopes the individual playground surfaces will cost 80 percent less than those with customary rubberized materials. Michael Kelly, park district CEO, acknowledges the city's priorities and choices as being cost-driven; the Park District will be heroic indeed if they pick a playground design that is equally inexpensive and exciting. The main point is that a major American city, strapped for financing, is reevaluating where they spend their funds, and they are not succumbing to the notion, supposedly based on safety, that bland rubber surfacing is a necessity.

On a national scale, some American nonprofits, including the TPL (with its wonderful motto, Great Parks = Great Cities), have just begun intergenerational initiatives; their Fitness Zones bring gym equipment to outside settings often next to playgrounds. Geared toward adults, these pieces of exercise equipment are meant to be free gyms. The Hayes Valley playground in San Francisco is one such example. The Fitness Zone overlooks the adjoining play space, and the results here, and elsewhere, show that the Fitness Zones are bringing teens—not just adults—into the parks. In some cases attendance went up 500 percent, and the degree of park use has risen overall. It is not a perfect intergenerational mix, but it is a powerful beginning.[24] Also heartening, TPL has begun to measure the "economic value" of urban parks, noting their effect on property costs, tourist dollars, and the overall well-being of local residents.

Changing our mindsets, institutions, and policies is just part of an equation of change. We have to contemplate what it would look like to alter our surroundings, to radically reconceptualize play sites. The next chapter provides a few superlative examples.

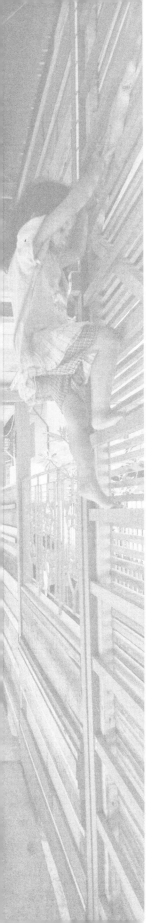

Conclusion | Paradigms

W E NEED TO RETHINK our approach to outdoor play spaces in order to revitalize them. In addition to insisting that play be child-initiated and child-directed, as play workers do, we need to demand sites that permit cautious risk taking, allow for failure and success, activate working memory, encourage problem solving, enhance friendships by being open and welcoming, and maybe include some vigorous aerobic exercise. We have already seen many examples of how this can be done.

We can continue a pioneering approach—and seek the best paradigms—if we concentrate on four scales for intervention: the street; the town square; the park; and the urban plan. We could also describe these same incursions as micro; multifunctional; magnetic; and comprehensive. In all the following cases, the intervention has stabilized or enhanced residential neighborhoods and improved how people experience their city. One of these examples (the first cited) could be adapted to include children; the three others, which already cater to mutli-age users, carry high costs—over $1 million—but each has used funds in a judicious way and has extracted the most possible number of uses for the money spent. All of these models reinterpret and expand, perhaps unknowingly, the small parks of Tokyo in the way they mesh with their environment, integrate children and adults of various ages, and encourage diverse populations to spend time together over the course of a day. They offer varying degrees of risk taking, succeeding and failing, employing EF, and exploring nature. The strongest thread that binds them is that they are all dynamic arenas where there is constant change and where visitors will never have the same experience twice.

1 | The City Street

Rebar Group is a multidisciplinary studio of artists that has been investigating "social furniture," the nexus of seating, playing, and improvising. They are thinking about how we could alter our permanent environment with spontaneous actions—or how spontaneity could offer clues to the best way to make things permanent. Bubbleware is one of their recent experi-

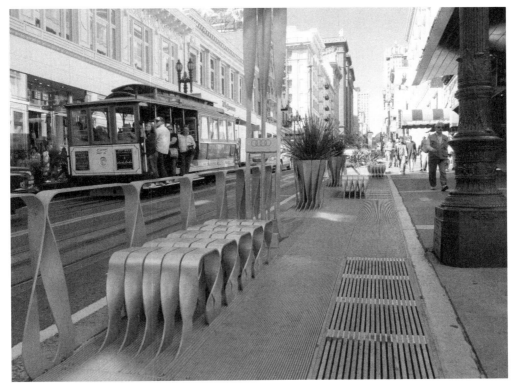

FIGURE C.1 | *Walter Hood, parklet on Powell Street (2010), San Francisco, California. Author's photograph, 2013.*

ments. It consists of three to ten core-strengthening exercise balls wrapped in a tough ballistic nylon. Bubbleware can be used for seating, jumping, or even as "movable parts." As Matt Passmore, one of the partners in Rebar explains, this very fluid movement allows users to find their most comfortable spots. It becomes a "prototyping" of urban space where the users, who have sanctioned and tested the product, inspire more permanent designs.

Rebar also explores leftover, underutilized spaces, "niche spaces" that have artistic and human potential.[1] The legacy of Aldo van Eyck continues in an altered form, although the Rebar artists also cite artist Gordon Matta-Clark as a forebear. Rebar has been particularly active in developing redundant space since 2005, when the group leased a single parking spot and transformed it into a tiny urban park, a PARKlet, for a day. Awareness of exploiting parking space caught on, and PARKing Day is now an annual worldwide event.[2]

With the success of the parklet, Rebar saw the potential to transform parking spaces into viable locations for adults. More than thirty-one are in place as semipermanent installations in Rebar's hometown of San Francisco. The city has a Pavement to Park program (under the aegis of the Planning Department) to issue permits. Different architects and designers have been able to put their imprint on built results that are showing up throughout the city. A restaurant, for instance, can construct a parklet at its curb as long as it makes the space available to anyone, not just its own customers. The startup cost is typically about $12,000; the annual fee to reserve two parking spots is $221.[3]

Rebar is considering how to extend the concept so that it might be large enough for family areas. Rebar's recent parklet inserted into a flatbed truck that had been broken apart, shortened, and then reassembled, might be a way to provide play space close to, yet slightly removed from, the street. A new parklet on both sides of Powell Street, along the path of a San Francisco cable car on the city's busiest thoroughfare, shows that some of the parklets that already exist are bringing together mixed ages groups; kids already see the potential for climbing. Landscape architect and sculptor Walter Hood (Hood Design) designed this extensive four-part parklet (with two sections on either side of Powell Street). Hood placed aluminum and wood grills on the expanded sidewalk and then designed aluminum street furniture and solar lights to spring from them. It shows that the parklet can be a barrier, keeping kids off the street, at the same time that young users can energize the street with their antics on whatever the parklet provides for climbing and jumping. There is plenty of space for older people to rest on stylized aluminum seating.[4]

2 | The City Square

Larger-scale interventions are effective when they transform underused, abandoned, or forsaken urban space into areas of activity for many age groups. These often fold play sites into grander environments that might include redirection of traffic, as well as new areas for recreation. The public art firm Carve worked with landscape architect Dijk & Co. and architects and designers, concrete to create Van Beuningenplein. The problem with this square (completed in 2011), in Amsterdam's West district, is that it does not photograph well. It is a significant achievement, a wide-ranging urban scheme whose scope and vitality are difficult to capture in an image or two.

The three-firm team worked together to blend what appear to be opposing needs: a youth center clubhouse, a sports facilities (soccer, skateboarding, basketball), a multi-age play site, a teen center, a separate building for a site manager, and a place for adults to relax. In order to make this

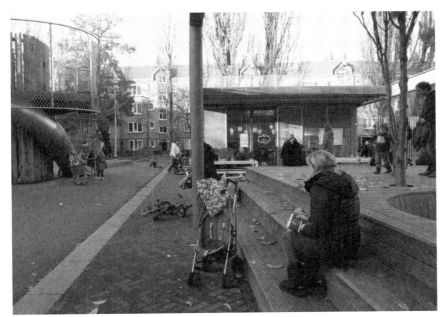

FIGURE C.2 | *Concrete Architects, Dijk & Co. landscape architects, and Carve; Van Beuningenplein (2011), Amsterdam, Netherlands. View toward the cafe. Author's photograph, 2012.*

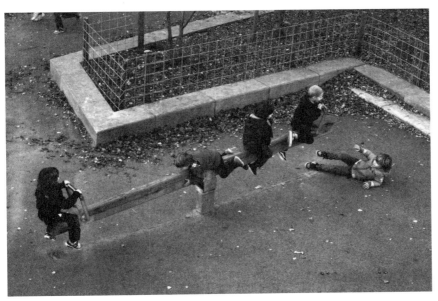

FIGURE C.3 | *Concrete Architects, Dijk & Co. landscape architects, and Carve; Van Beuningenplein (2011), Amsterdam, Netherlands. Author's photograph, 2012.*

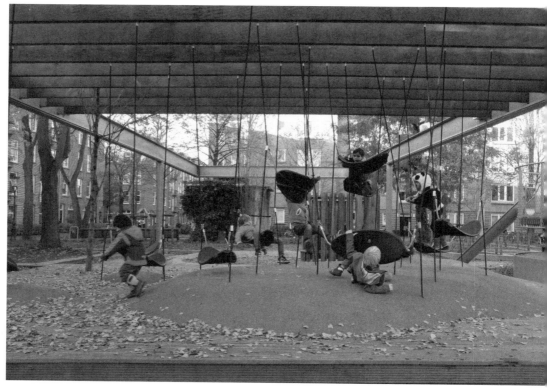

FIGURE C.4 | *Concrete Architects, Dijk & Co. landscape architects, and Carve; Van Beuningenplein (2011), Amsterdam, Netherlands. Carve designed this ingenious climbing device by reconfiguring sling swings. Author's photograph, 2012. (Plate 11)*

a community space with as many amenities as possible, the municipality decided to place all parking underground. The hefty price of €7 million has to be seen in terms of digging out and creating underground parking and rebuilding and revitalizing an entire square.[5]

Before the new construction, the site was both derelict and a blank slate filled with potential. It was an empty asphalt surface with no reminder that there had been playgrounds here as early as 1915. The surrounding housing, built in the 1930s, remained in excellent condition. As part of the project, greenery of trees and bushes now enclose the space. It is lush but porous. There are no gates and no signs to prevent anyone from entering. The neighborhood, once considered rough, has been revitalized by this new community resource that attracts visitors, day or night.

The architects, concrete, organized the space into three distinct rooms; twelve-foot-high steel beams, which contain computerized colored lighting, reinforce the distinctions. The main entrance, on the east, has a glass-enclosed teen center with a panna pitch on the roof. This area also has the sports sections: one that is loosely constructed for soccer, and the other for basketball. The edges permit skateboarding. The center "room" is dedicated to picnic seating, a stage with a sunken area for trees, and another free-standing pavilion. The seating is located so that adults can see children in both directions but are at a sensible, nonintrusive distance. The pavilion, originally intended for a site manager, became vacant after the position was eliminated; it is now a thriving restaurant. The combination of lighting, seating, and cafe means that adults are welcome to come and gather in the evenings. The cafe, whose walls can pivot open during warm months, remains open for dinner twice a week.

The last room—the one on the western side—is dedicated to play. Carve has come up with ingenious devices. They designed the old-fashioned seesaw as well as a sand area; broad, low seating platforms; and two climbers. One low climber has a metal ladder at the right height for a toddler, who can climb to a surface where it is possible to run around a tree and then exit via a fairly steep metal slide. Older children can go to the larger climber, where the rungs of the ladder make it clear that kids have to be five or six to attempt this.[6] They can ascend to a wavy platform and even dip into baskets that let them be suspended above the playground floor.

For a swinging and climbing structure, Carve devised a sensational (and very inexpensive!) amalgamation of both. They took swing slings, suspended them from wooden beams that intersect with the steel frame, and created an entirely new piece of equipment. The slings are densely packed and at different heights. Children can swing on one, either high or low to the ground, or they can climb from one to another. It takes perseverance, awareness of height, and agility in moving. Each child determines his own level of competence and risk, with the possibility of taking a harder and more difficult path each time it's tried. The rubberized material below is mounded into a single hill with some lower hills nearby. These provide visual interest in addition to protection.

Van Beuningenplein demonstrates why we should put money into public space: it has revitalized a section of the city; it brings all types of people together; and it has different populations at different times, including toddlers in the morning, older kids in the afternoon, and adults in the evening. It demonstrates, too, that sports clubs and organized activities can share space with more casual visitors of varying ages, including young children.

3 | The City Park

The city park is the usual scale and place where we expect play to occur. The Helen Diller Playground at Dolores Park in San Francisco shows how design can be done exquisitely, thereby making a contribution to the beauty of the city (which is already considerable) and retention of families in the neighborhood. The proponents—which included a local friends group, a San Francisco philanthropist, and the Recreation and Park Department—wanted to make sure that this part of the city contained a mix of residents, including young families, in this gentrifying area close to the Mission district.[7] A skilled landscape architect, Steven Koch (Koch Landscape Architecture), has created a space (completed in 2012) that fits easily into the rest of the park while taking advantage of a sublime site overlooking the city.[8]

This is a public-private venture, one that grew out of a local, modest endeavor to fix drainage on an old playground. Nancy Madynski, a general contractor, lived in the area. She had grown up nearby (as one of ten chil-

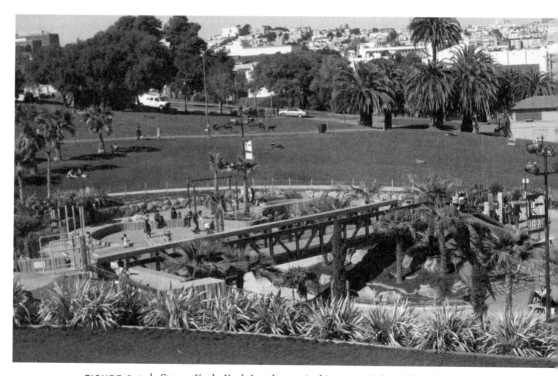

FIGURE C.5 | *Steven Koch, Koch Landscape Architecture, Helen Diller Playground at Dolores Park (2012), San Francisco, California. The playground fits into the deep bowl of the park and is hardly visible to cars passing by on the street. Author's photograph, 2013. (Plate 12)*

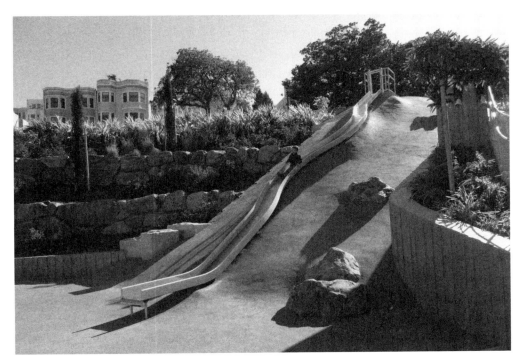

FIGURE C.6 | *Steven Koch, Koch Landscape Architecture, Helen Diller Playground at Dolores Park (2012), San Francisco, California. The stone wall is beautiful and very climbable. Author's photograph, 2013.*

dren) and has fond childhood memories of rolling down the park's steep hills when she was a child and knowing it was time to go home when the street lights went on (not unlike the way kids now respond to clock chimes that ring in Tokyo parks). Her original plan was to ask some contractor friends to spend a morning fixing the flooding. She found, however, that a web of rules and regulations prevailed; these intercepted her intentions before anything could happen.

This one small gesture started a groundswell. Over a five-year period, Madynski and fellow residents formed a Friends of Dolores Park Playground organization; forged a relationship with the San Francisco Parks Alliance; and welcomed funding from local philanthropist Jackie Safier, who donated half of the required $3.5 million in honor of her mother, Helen Diller. All three of the leaders—Safier, Madynski, and Phil Ginsburg, the general manager of the Recreation and Park Department—knew that they wanted a distinctive play space, one that was not a coop filled with cookie-cutter equipment. Safier, in particular, insisted that there be nighttime lighting so that there would be extensive use at all hours of the day. She also

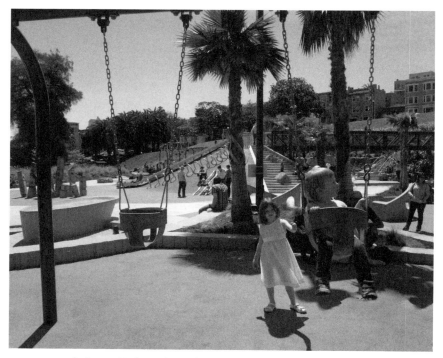

FIGURE C.7 | *Steven Koch, Koch Landscape Architecture, Helen Diller Playground at Dolores Park (2012), San Francisco, California. The Koch-designed sand boat, which can be accessible to wheelchairs, is in the left middle background; the bridge and slide can be seen at the back right. Author's photograph, 2013.*

contended that the playground should have both play and aesthetic significance, so that it would be enhancing to people's daily lives. She wants to see this neighborhood have vibrant public resources that might add reasons for families to remain in the city.

Koch's plan takes advantage of the site, a deep bowl. He stayed within the same square footage as earlier playground iterations (the site has housed a playground since the 1940s or 1950s), but he pushed the playground against the rim of the bowl so that he could exploit the height. He placed a series of terraced quarter- to three-ton boulders along the side as a retaining wall. Koch arranged additional plantings along the stone walls. The high stone walls, in conjunction with the deep bowl, create an embracing perimeter. It is possible to have no fencing (although this decision was controversial in the neighborhood). Koch used a low, concrete serpentine wall along the entrance side, at grade with the rest of Dolores Park. The wall is suitable for seating but is not intrusive; it, too, contributes to a loosely defined edge. Kids are protected by this single entrance and the fact that even a small child "on the run" could not go too far along the park's vast rolling lawn. Without fencing, the playground blends into the park site and extends a relaxed welcome in place of the standard barrier fence. Koch says that he hopes to evoke — but not copy — some of the elements (serpentine wall, mounds, and bridges) that remain distinctive in Richard Dattner's playgrounds in New York City. Koch's keen sense of history links this playground to Dattner and, by extension, to the Kahn-Noguchi playground that Dattner admired. Like the unbuilt Kahn-Noguchi plan, Koch's scheme nestles into the ground and is not really seen from the street view.

The stone terracing is not without playability. Since the walls and foliage are high and daunting, they are a challenge, even a magnet, to an active child. Even six- and seven-year-olds try to figure out how to secure their feet on the rocks so that they can get to the plants, and then try to reach the second tier. There is no clear path to success; each child has to make his own choices to have the triumph of getting to the highest level.

Koch designed some pieces of climbing equipment, including a wooden tower and a stone wall with a short tunnel. Neither piece guarantees a successful climb; children have to work hard by planning their moves and judging how much to attempt. In contrast, the tunnel opening in the stone has become a tiny protected space where kids come to relax and chat. Koch also added a super slide to allow kids to experience speed and thrills. His is a wavy embankment version, one that pays homage to several concrete embankment slides that this city forged in the 1970s.[9] By being narrow and high, the piece gives kids a sense of doing something perilous.

Koch also designed the elliptical sand pit. A raised portion resembles a boat (there used to be a pond in the park); it is a sculptural addition that also shows that a "sand table" for kids in wheelchairs can be functional and elegant. The "sand boat" is a place for parents to hold little kids or for toddlers to explore. Nearby, "waves," or low hills, in the unitary surfacing provide visual interest as well as another low obstacle course for little kids.

4 | The Urban Plan

With five lanes of traffic on each side of the polluted Manzanares River, the Madrid Rio site did not seem a likely play environment. A series of transformative events led to play sites that now figure prominently in this multimillion-dollar project to redesign an entire section of Madrid, Spain. The mayor of Madrid (Alberto Ruiz Gallardon) initiated the project in 2004, calling for placing underground the highway that had divided the western part of the city from the center of Madrid. Once the tunnel project was complete, the mayor called for a competition (2008) to enhance the resulting surface spaces that emerged and to integrate land on both sides of the water The nearby densely packed western apartments, which date from the 1950s and were sometimes only 100 feet from the riverbank, had few amenities to draw people out of their apartments. Playgrounds in other areas of the city were usually geared only to small children. Therefore, the goal was not only to blend poor neighborhoods into the general fold of the city but also to provide the type of public space that these neighborhoods lacked and supplement the experiences for people coming from other parts of town.

Four combined firms — Burgos & Garrido/Porras La-Casta/Rubio & Alvarez Sala/West 8 under the direction of Ginés Garrido — won the competition.[10] The successful scheme (completed in 2011, just before the worst of the financial crisis began) activates the river by creating new foot bridges, and adding recreational activities along both shores. There are skateboarding sites, paths for walking and jogging, and picnic areas. The play spaces — a total of fifteen — are particularly noteworthy. They pop up suddenly on both sides of the river, small intrusions that are part of the flow of leisure activities. They offer places to stop or take on new challenges. There are plenty of amenities for adults, but it is clear that this urban design aspires to bring children and teens into the daily mix. There is no fencing, so play areas sometimes abut cafes and are always close to walking paths. One of the architects who worked on the project tells a revealing anecdote about a moment soon after the park opened: he came and took pictures of teens who were playing there, although these youngsters were worried that he would call the police who would throw them out. These teens hadn't yet realized that this space was meant for them, and they were using it in a suitable way.

The designers, who conceived each riverbank separately, set out to evoke the memories of a child in rural Spain of the past. They decided on recalling the forest and the riverbed. The west side evokes the forest and represents the north of the country, the source of the Manzanares River. The designers interpreted the forest as burned or destroyed. Pine trees, as irregular as possible, stand in for ruined timberland. German manufacturer Richter Spielgeräte provided most of the play equipment, using their signature robinia wood structures to blend with the nearby pines. By grouping similar activities together, such as a field of horizontal climbers or a separate expanse of vertical poles, these play areas (eleven on this side) have a haunting beauty. On several of the climbers, children have to be aware of the swaying

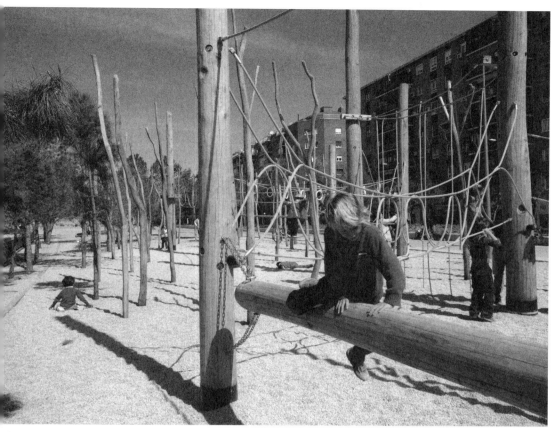

FIGURE C.8 | *Burgos & Garrido/Porras La Casta/Rubio & Álvarez-Sala/West 8; Team Director: Ginés Garrido, Madrid Rio (2011), Madrid, Spain. This is one of several play areas in the Salon de Pinos. Courtesy of Richter Spielgeräte.*

as they try to climb up. In other areas, kids have to maneuver their way among dense poles that are actually a maze, so they are unable to calculate a route in advance. The pea-gravel surface is subtle; it does not scream for attention.

In one area, under a footbridge, very long swings attract older children. Dutch landscape architects West 8 painted bright red circles under the bridge and then suspended the swings from these "bulls eyes." The use of leftover space and seamless connection to its surroundings call forth the work of their compatriot predecessor, Aldo van Eyck.

The eastern side of the river—the Arganzuela section, which recalls the dry riverbeds of southern Spain—has fewer play areas. It is denser and more compact, and often covered with stone-filled dry creeks. One major play feature is a slide hill. West 8 designed the hill and the plantings. Richter custom designed the eight slides that have unusual sizes and angles in order to give the most thrilling sensations. The success of this entire project, and specifically this hill slide, was evident after the first week of use. There were so many active children and they were so eager to try each slide that they jammed the area and trampled the foliage. The flexible attitude of West 8 can be seen in how they then reconstructed the hill. They made the concrete steps and terracing more irregular and less predictable. Children will have to think more about how to approach the slides. The change will force them to slow down and consider their best way to continue up the hill. West 8 also came up with planting that is less dense and more hearty, better resistant to destruction. It is to West 8's credit that they transformed the entire site into an interactive, thought-provoking piece of "equipment." They added a nice local reference by incorporating pieces of an old nearby fountain into the concrete terracing. The park's chief accomplishment can be seen on a summer evening. As the day cools off, the park becomes a retreat for varied populations who relax, eat, and play. They can stay as long as they want and often remain until late in the evening.

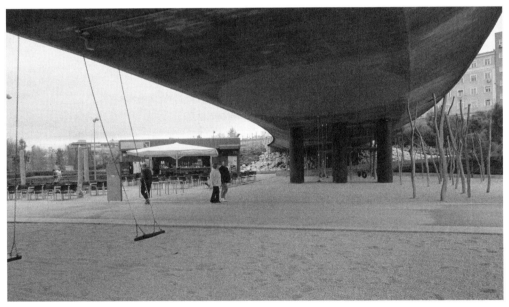

FIGURE C.9 | *Burgos & Garrido/Porras La Casta/Rubio & Álvarez-Sala/West 8; Team Director: Ginés Garrido, Madrid Rio (2011), Madrid, Spain. The swings, suspended from a red bullseye under the bridge, evoke Aldo van Eyck's use of "leftover" spaces to support activities for children. This view also shows how other play areas, a cafe, and a walking, jogging trail are interwoven seamlessly. Photograph by Robert S. Solomon, 2013. (Plate 13)*

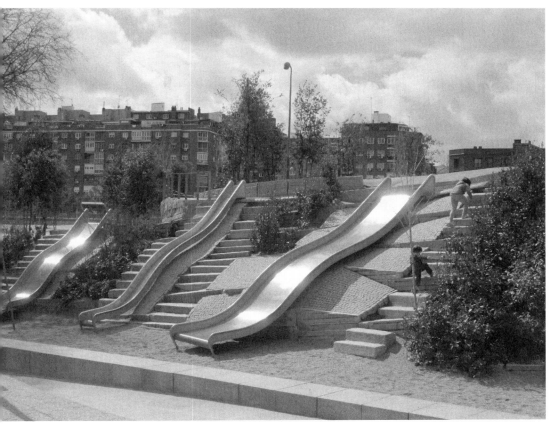

FIGURE C.10 | *Burgos & Garrido/Porras La Casta/Rubio & Álvarez-Sala/West 8; Team Director: Ginés Garrido, Madrid Rio (2011), Madrid, Spain. These are three of the eight slides on the "slide hill" of the Arganzuela side. Courtesy of Richter Spielgeräte.*

Inspiration

These four examples—from San Francisco, Amsterdam, and Madrid —should inspire us to think differently about play sites. We see a variety of intrusions on different scales, and carrying different price tags. We also see how visionary individuals—local leaders, donors, patrons, municipal administrators—were able to act valiantly and create specific successes that include children but extend the notion of a play site. These ensembles, which fit seamlessly into neighborhoods, include the possibility of bringing everyone—not just children—together. Paige Johnson, the intelligent and perceptive founder of the Playscapes blog, asks correctly if we might have entered a "post-playground era."[11]

Wake Up America

Americans who feel passionately about play are often like comedian Stephen Colbert when he says that "American Exceptionalism" is the belief we are always right. It is time to look around. We are an extraordinary country, but, when it comes to play sites, we are not advanced. We are far behind many other parts of the world; we lag very significantly behind the British on evaluating risk, and we trail many Europeans and the Japanese in creative design solutions. We have been spending a lot of money on ideas that are old; we repeat tired models, keep to the same formulas, and do not actively pursue change.

Now is the time for inventive attitudes and achievements. We need new visions of possibilities, especially at a national level, so that people who commission playgrounds — a group that includes parents, school districts, and parks departments — will have support to insist on better outcomes. We should spend less money; we should find ways to repurpose or adapt redundant materials. There is a lesson in the old sewer culvert (about three feet high and ten feet long) at the Bay Area Discovery Museum; it was left over from construction and is now a successful (cleaned and painted) place for running and hiding because the staff recognized the play potential of refuse.

We have to evaluate designs and see what they offer children. Are these sites that foster risk taking, succeeding and failing, planning or using working memory? We have to support kids' independence. Responsive design will not produce an area where kids will learn all their life skills, but it can reinforce and support scientific research in hopes that children are spending time in places that could help them thrive.

We can look to our future by taking note of the past, especially the year 1968, which is known best for protests and assassinations. We should also be aware of a quieter, double-edged revolution that was trying to invigorate public space for children. Alfred Ledermann and Alfred Trachsel, Swiss authors, came out with the second edition of their book *Creative Playgrounds and Recreation Centers.*[12] In the same year, Lady Allen of Hurtwood published her fifth book, *Planning for Play*. These books, both of which try to energize how we create public spaces for children, start from diametrically opposed premises. Ledermann and Trachsel present images of successful, innovative play spaces. If we can put aside the telltale clothing and hair styles, we could argue that most of their examples are illustrations of the type of spaces to which we aspire: very high, thrill-inducing slides, enormous challenging logs to climb, large water areas in which to frolic. They look to what had been accomplished, particularly in Europe, and they celebrate it.

Lady Allen, on the other hand, sounds an alarm. She already senses changes are afoot and these will result in further weakening of exciting play spaces. She presciently asks, "Why are so many of the new playgrounds stagnant?"[13] She decries fixed equipment, ordered from catalogs, that sits on an antiseptic "stark desert of hard surfacing."[14] And she warns against overly designed unique playgrounds that can be expensive and equally dull.[15] She sees how local authorities dumb down play so that they don't have to deal with insurance issues.[16] She recognizes that there is great confusion for everyone and that in the design world, "Architects pick up bit and piece from here and there, and fit the children into the playground, rather than the reverse."[17] And she had the guts to say, "A playground that is not attractive to children is a waste of land and money."[18] She even saw how the overprotection of parents was keeping children from being independent.[19] Unknowingly, she foretold our current afflictions while Ledermann and Trachsel, also unknowingly, supplied answers.

The year 1968 was a watershed. England and America continued the restricted positions that Lady Allen enumerated. We have seen how England, in the past two decades, has begun to alter its stance while we continue down a narrowing path of fear and overprotectivness. We need to stop and think. It should be our calling to respond to Lady Allen's perceptions by eliminating the constraints she identified and that have become even more imposing obstacles since her time. Our plan should be to vanquish (finally) Lady Allen's fears and have playgrounds that are as exciting and stimulating as the ones the Swiss authors highlighted.

The playground is an undervalued resource. We have to readjust our thinking, seeing it as a vital community space. Pediatrician Robert Whitaker suggests the metaphor of "a sanctuary" to describe an ideal playground.[20] If we rethink what kids need and where they can take advantage of activities that enhance their overall well-being, perhaps we can provide play sites that are sanctuaries: safe, welcoming, inspiring, supportive, and friendly environments that sit seamlessly within a greater urban landscape.[21]

Notes

Introduction

1. Fergus P. Hughes, *Children, Play, and Development*, 4th ed. (Los Angeles, CA: Sage, 2010), 4–5.

2. Jacky Kilvington and Ali Wood, *Reflective Playwork* (London: Continuum International, 2010), 17–18.

3. Ellen Beate Hansen Sandseter, "Characteristics of Risky Play," *Journal of Adventure Education and Outdoor Learning* 9, no. 1 (2009): 3; Peter K. Smith, *Children and Play* (Malden, MA: Wiley-Blackwell, 2010), 6–10. Smith, reporting on his own research and building on work that L. Krasnor and D. Pepler published in 1980, defines play as enjoyable behavior that is intrinsically motivated, nonliteral, flexible, and more concerned with means than ends.

4. Kilvington and Wood, *Reflective Playwork*, 18. See also M. Conway, "The Playwork Principles," in *Foundations of Playwork*, ed. F. Brown and C. Taylor (Maidenhead: Open University Press, 2008). Kilvington and Wood, 28, report that in the 1980s, a movement in the United Kingdom attempted to tie play with child development. It was called SPICE, for "social interaction; physical activity; intellectual stimulation; creative achievement; and emotional stability," but it became so narrow that it created "over-structured ways of planning for play."

5. Smith, *Children and Play*, 213.

6. Stuart Brown's National Institute of Play, alluded to in Anthony D. Pellegrini, "Research and Policy on Children's Play," *Child Development Perspectives* 3, no 2 (2009): 131–36. For Brown's views, see Stuart Brown and Christopher Vaughan, *Play! How It Shapes the Brain, Opens the Mind, and Invigorates the Soul* (New York: Penguin, 2009). Peter Gray makes an even more outrageous assertion in his "The Decline of Play and the Rise of Psychopathology in Children and Adolescents," *American Journal of Play* 4, no. 3 (2011). Gray acknowledges that "correlation, of course does not prove causation," even though he tries hard to link these phenomena. Without ruling out factors that might have caused psychopathology, Gray can make only limited guesses.

We should also be wary of blaming lack of play for the late maturation of young adults: the MacArthur Foundation has shown that economic factors and other social causes have been the primary cause. "Young people are now much more aware of what it takes to be autonomous, and they tend to be disinclined to take on commitments that they cannot honor." See Frank F. Furstenberg, Jr., Ruben G. Rumbaut, and Richard A. Settersten Jr., "On the Frontier of Adulthood: Emerging Themes and New Directions," in their book of the same title (Chicago: University of Chicago Press, 2005), 6.

7. Pellegrini, "Research and Policy on Children's Play," 131–36.

8. Judy Dunn, *Children's Friendships: The Beginnings of Intimacy* (Malden, MA: Blackwell, 2004), 30.

9. Anthony D. Pellegrini, "Rough-and-Tumble Play from Childhood through

Adolescence," in *Introduction to Play from Birth to Twelve: Contexts, Perspectives, and Meanings*, 2nd ed., ed. Doris Pronin Fromberg and Doris Bergen (New York: Routledge, 2006), 111.

10. Anthony D. Pellegrini, *The Role of Play in Human Development* (Oxford: Oxford University Press, 2009), 199–200.

11. Smith, Children and Play, 197.

12. Stuart Lester and Wendy Russell, *Play England: Play for a Change: Play, Policy and Practice: A Review of Contemporary Perspectives* (London: National Children's Bureau, 2008), ch. 3. In 2000, the Children's Play Council, the predecessor to Play England, published a report, *Making the Case for Play: Gathering the Evidence*. The authors, Issy Cole-Hamilton, Andrew Harrop, and Cathy Street, concluded that "the *evidence* for the benefits of play is complex, often inconclusive, and there are a number of areas where data is seriously lacking and research is needed" (91).

13. The role of neuroscience in understanding daily behavior is currently under reevaluation. Mike Anderson and Sergio Della Sala make the case for cognitive psychology's being the field that "does all the useful work or 'heavy lifting.'" See Anderson and Della Sala, *Neuroscience in Education: The Good, the Bad, and the Ugly* (Oxford ScholarshipOnline, available at http://www.oxfordscholarship .com/view/10.1093/acprof:oso/9780199600496 .001.0001/acprof-9780199600496, accessed May 2012). *New York Times* political columnist David Brooks notes that he set out to write a book about neuroscience but ended up writing a book about psychology: *The Social Animal: The Hidden Sources of Love, Character, and Achievement* (New York: Random House, 2011). See also Walter Mischel and David Brooks, "The News from Psychological Science: A Conversation between David Brooks and Walter Mischel," *Perspectives on Psychological Science* 6 (2011): 515.

14. Alison Gopnik, *The Philosophical Baby: What Children's Minds Tell Us about Truth, Love,* *and the Meaning of Life* (New York: Picador, 2009), 12.

15. Jack P. Shonkoff and Deborah A. Phillips, eds., *From Neurons to Neighborhoods: The Science of Early Childhood Development* (Washington, DC: National Academy Press, 2000), 23.

16. Foresters, press release, November 16, 2013. "Foresters, KaBOOM! & Volunteers Revitalize Columbia Community with New Playground." The actual quotation, alluding to Foresters support of playgrounds since 2006 and repeated in other press material from them is: "Over their 15 year lifespan, these playgrounds will provide more than 2.6 million children and their families with an opportunity to spend quality time together." Even some of the most refined and well-crafted pieces may have just a twenty-year life if they are well cared for. Peter Heuken (Director of Projects, Richter Spielgeräte GmbH), email to author, December 11, 2013. He notes that fifteen years is the standard in the industry.

17. Rhonda Clements, "An Investigation of the Status of Outdoor Play," *Contemporary Issues in Early Childhood* 5, no. 1 (2004): 68–80.

18. Tim Waller et al., "The Dynamics of Early Childhood Spaces: Opportunities for Outdoor Play?" *European Early Childhood Education Research Journal* 18, no. 4 (2010): 440.

19. Hillary L. Burdette and Robert C. Whitaker, "Resurrecting Free Play in Young Children: Looking beyond Fitness and Fatness to Attention, Affiliation, and Affect," *Archives of Pediatric & Adolescent Medicine* 159 (2005): 46–50. Unstructured play dropped 25 percent for American children between 1981 and 1997.

20. PLANyc is a massive twenty-seven-year agenda for saving energy and improving the quality of life in New York City. One goal is to provide a park within a ten-minute walk of every New York resident. In 2007 there were 290 closed schoolyards in areas with insufficient parks. PLANyc opened sixty-nine immediately, then formed a partnership with the Trust for Public Land to improve

and open the remaining sites. Most of these transformations were completed by 2013. For further information and the most recent updates, see www.nyc.gov/html/planyc2030 /html/theplan/public-spaces.shtml. It is worth noting a historic precedent. Robert Moses was a proponent of developing schoolyards with public parks in the 1930s. See Rachel Iannacone, "Neighborhood Playgrounds and Parks," in *Robert Moses and the Modern City: The Transformation of New York*, ed. Hilary Ballon and Kenneth T. Jackson (New York: W. W. Norton, 2007), 174. For more information on ways to achieve joint use, see California Pan-Ethnic Health Network, "Unlocking the Playground: Achieving Equity in Physical Activity Spaces," a 2009 report on a series of forums, at www.cpehn.org:pdfs.

21. Amy F. Ogata, *Designing the Creative Child: Playthings and Places in Midcentury America* (Minneapolis: University of Minnesota Press, 2013), 8.

22. Daily Mail on Line, http://www.dailymail .co.uk/news/article-2275593/Playground -Corinium-Via-estate-Cotswolds-closed -complained-bright.html, February 8, 2013. Neighbors in the housing estate, Corinium Via, deemed the equipment "too bright"; developers closed the playground until the issue was resolved.

23. Kenneth R. Ginsburg, "The Importance of Play in Promoting Healthy Child Development and Maintaining Strong Parent-Child Bonds," *Pediatrics* 119, no. 1 (January 2007): 182–88; Regina M. Milteer and Kenneth R. Ginsburg, "The Importance of Play in Promoting Healthy Child Development and Maintaining Strong Parent-Child Bond: Focus on Children in Poverty," *Pediatrics* 129, no. 1 (December 2011): 204–13.

24. Elger Blitz of Carve supplied information about this project via e-mail to author, September 30, 2013.

25. Ibid., October 25, 2013. The cost was less than $220,000.

26. E-mail, Elger Blitz of Carve to author, September 30, 2013.

27. S. Rogers and J. Evans, "Playing the Games: Exploring Role Play from Children's Perspectives," *European Early Childhood Education Research Journal* 14, no. 1 (2006): 43–56, quoted in Helen Tovey, *Playing Outdoors: Spaces and Places, Risk and Challenge* (New York: McGraw Hill, 2007), 18.

28. Robin Marantz Henig, "Taking Play Seriously," *New York Times Magazine*, February 17, 2008.

29. Kristen L. Knutson and Even Van Cauter, "Association between Sleep Loss and Increased Risk of Obesity and Diabetes," *Annals of the New York Academy of Sciences* 1129 (2008): 287–304. This is just one of the more fascinating reports that highlights the complexity of the obesity issue. Apparently loss of sleep exacerbates loss of the hormone that regulates a feeling of satiation and increases the hormone that raises feelings of hunger. For bullying, see Emily Bazelon, *Sticks and Stones: Defeating the Culture of Bullying and Rediscovering the Power of Character and Empathy* (New York: Random House, 2013). Developmental psychologist Helene Guldberg has written about the positive aspects of bullying in her *Reclaiming Childhood: Freedom and Play in an Age of Fear* (London: Routledge, 2009).

30. Henig, "Taking Play Seriously," notes that *The Dangerous Book for Boys* was on the bestseller list for the previous nine months.

31. Aase Eriksen, *Playground Design: Outdoor Environments for Learning and Development* (New York: Van Nostrand Reinhold Company, 1985), ix–5.

32. Ibid.

1. The Problem

1. Amy Ogata, "Creative Playthings: Educational Toys and Postwar American Culture," *Winterthur Portfolio* 39, no. 2/3 (2004): 141.

2. I thank Tim Gill (www

.rethinkingchildhood.com) for pointing this out to me.

3. Judith Warner, *Perfect Madness: Motherhood in the Age of Anxiety* (New York: Riverhead Books, 2005), 91–98.

4. Shirley Wyver et al., "Ten Ways to Restrict Children's Freedom to Play: The Problem of Surplus Safety," *Contemporary Issues in Early Childhood* 11, no. 3 (2010): 270; Marianne B. Staempfli, "Reintroducing Adventure into Children's Outdoor Play Environments," *Environment and Behavior* 41 (2009): 275.

5. Architect Richard Dattner has often been quoted regarding how kids — or their parents — invoke lawyers. Most recently he was cited in Carol Kino's piece "The Work behind Child's Play," *New York Times*, July 3, 2013.

6. Just a few states have adopted the guidelines into state legislation. Teri Hendy, telephone interview with author, May 8, 2013.

7. Ibid.

8. Ellen Beate Hansen Sandseter and Leif Edward Ottesen Kennair, "Children's Risky Play from an Evolutionary Perspective: The Anti-Phobic Effects of Thrilling Experiences," *Evolutionary Psychology* 9, no. 2 (2011): 260–61.

9. Helle Nebelong, interview with author, December 14, 2011, Copenhagen.

10. Sandra Aamodt and Sam Wang, *Welcome to Your Child's Brain* (New York: Bloomsbury, 2011), 129.

11. Edward F. Zigler and Sandra J. Bishop-Josef, "The Cognitive Child versus the Whole Child: Lessons from 40 Years of Head Start," in *Play=Learning: How Play Motivates and Enhances Children's Cognitive and Social-Emotional Growth*, ed. Dorothy G. Singer, Roberta Michnick Golinkoff, and Kathy Hirsh-Pasek (New York: Oxford University Press, 2006), 23.

12. Elena Bodrova and Deborah J. Leong, *Tools of the Mind: The Vygotskian Approach to Early Childhood Education*, 2nd ed. (Upper Saddle River, NJ: Pearson/Merrill Prentice Hall, 2007), 6–8.

13. Ogata, "Creative Playthings," 135. In the 1950s, manufacturers such as Playskool and Holgate segregated their catalogs according to age.

14. John Medina, *Brain Rules for Baby: How to Raise a Smart and Happy Child from Zero to Five* (Seattle: Pear, 2010), 154.

15. Greet Cardon et al., "The Contribution of Preschool Playground Factors in Explaining Children's Physical Activity during Recess," *International Journal of Behavioral Nutrition and Physical Activity* 5, no. 11 (2008).

16. Jay Beckwith, interview with author, May 7, 2012, Novato, CA.

17. "2008 Physical Activity Guidelines for Americans," www.health.gov/PAGuidelines/pdf/PAguide.pdf. To be fair, the guidelines do include "playground equipment" in their list of activities to develop muscles. They presumably mean something like monkey bars. They also suggest climbing trees and playing tug of war.

18. Jackie Safier (donor of Helen Diller Playground), interview with author, February 25, 2013, San Francisco.

19. Tanya Byron, address to North of England Education Conference, "Mind, Brain, Community: Inspiring Learners, Strengthening Resilience," January 16–18, 2013, at Sheffield Hallam University, reported by Richard Garner, "Children Brought up 'In Captivity' by Risk Adverse Parents, Says Leading Child Psychologist," *Independent*, January 18, 2013.

20. Linda Pollak, interview with author, April 22, 2013, New York City. Pollak and her partner Sandro Marpillero took advantage of fencing that would have been too expensive to tear down by creating a seating area with plantings and a trellis. The site is the learning garden at the Whitestone Branch of the Queens (NY) Public Library (2010).

21. Steven Mintz, *Huck's Raft: A History of American Childhood* (Cambridge: Belknap Press of Harvard University Press, 2004), 337–40.

22. Ibid., 339.

23. Sarah Knight, "Forest School: Playing on the Wild Side," in *The Excellence of Play*,

3rd ed., ed. Janet Moyles (Berkshire, UK: Open University Press, 2010), 190.

24. According to the National Center for Missing and Exploited Children (www .missingkids.com), 1999 is the last year for which abduction statistics were gathered. The Missing Children's Act of 1982 allowed data on missing children to be entered into the National Crime Information Center of the FBI.

25. Justine Taylor, "An Examination of Media Accounts of Child Abductions in the United States," master's thesis, Pennsylvania State University, 2010.

26. Daniel Gardner, *The Science of Fear: How the Culture of Fear Manipulates Your Brain* (New York: Plume Books, 2009), 185–86.

27. Bill Durodié, "Fear of Adults Has Devastating Effects for Kids; Efforts to Keep Children Safe Often End up with Negative Repercussions," *Times-Colonist* (Victoria, British Columbia), August 15, 2012.

28. Wyver et al., "Ten Ways," 264.

29. Robert C. Whitaker, telephone interview with author, February 26, 2013.

30. These figures come from an opinion poll commissioned by Playday 2010, a massive public event for play awareness. Play England coordinates Playday with Play Scotland, Play Wales, and Playboard Northern Ireland.

31. Isami Kinoshita, professor of environmental science and landscape architecture, Chiba University, interview with author, May 24, 2013, Tokyo.

32. Kenneth R. Ginsburg with Martha M. Jablow, *Building Resilience in Children and Teens: Giving Kids Roots and Wings*, 2nd ed. (Elk Grove Village, IL: American Academy of Pediatrics, 2011), 131.

33. Ray Oldenburg, *The Great Good Place* (Cambridge: Da Capo, 1989).

34. Eric Klinenberg, "Adaptation: How Can Cities Be 'Climate-proof'?" *New Yorker*, January 7, 2013, 32–37.

35. The estimate of the Association of Play Industries is that the cost of the surfacing can increase the budget by 40 percent. Teri Hendy, playground consultant, says that she has seen many instances where the cost of the poured-in-place rubber is the same as the cost of the equipment. Hendy, telephone interview with author, May 8, 2013.

36. David J. Ball, "Policy Issues and Risk-Benefit Trade Offs of 'Safer Surfacing' for Children's Playgrounds," *Accident Analysis and Prevention* 36, no. 4 (July 2004): 661–70, 668.

37. David J. Ball, "Trends in Fall Injuries Associated with Children's Outdoor Climbing Frames," *International Journal of Injury Control and Safety Promotion* 14, no. 1 (2007): 49–53.

38. CPSC, "Public Playground Safety Handbook," August 2012, 8–10.

39. David Spease, summary of research, forwarded by Teri Hendy in an e-mail to author, May 8, 2013.

40. I am grateful to Peter Heuken and Sharon Gamson Danks for pointing this out.

41. Wyver et al., "Ten Ways," 269.

42. I thank Nicky Washida for pointing this out to me.

43. Ian Frazier, "Muddy," in "Talk of the Town," *New Yorker*, December 10, 2012, 31–32. Frasier describes the Merrell Down & Dirty National Mud and Obstacle Series. During these 5k and 10k races, some fifty-six hundred people confront the obstacles on the course, including wading through a mud pool.

44. Ellen Beate Hansen Sandseter, interview with author, November 8, 2012, Trondheim, Norway.

45. Mary Ruebush, *Why Dirt Is Good: 5 Ways to Make Germs Our Friends* (New York: Kaplan, 2009), 36–37.

46. Ibid., 103. It is still unclear if Ruebush's idea, known more generally as the "hygiene hypothesis" and developed by others in the late 1980s, is completely accurate when it posits that lack of exposure to dirt may account for an uptick in allergies or even depression. We do know, however, that, because of cultural mores, girls are less likely to get dirty; this might

account for their higher prevalence of immune system diseases. See Sharyn Clough, "Gender and the Hygiene Hypothesis," *Social Science and Medicine* 30 (2010): 1–8.

47. Jane E. Brody, "Babies Know: A Little Dirt Is Good for You," *New York Times*, January 26, 2009.

48. Dr. Joel V. Weinstock, quoted in ibid.

49. Craig Anderson, "Comment," *Brainerd Dispatch*, March 10, 2013; another commenter in the same paper said she requested daily cleaning only for indoor playgrounds.

50. Paula S. Fass, "The Child-Centered Family? New Rules in Postwar America," in *Reinventing Childhood after World War II*, ed. Paula Fass and Michael Grossberg (Philadelphia: University of Pennsylvania Press, 2011), 16–17.

51. Joy Hendry, *Understanding Japanese Society*, 4th ed. (New York: Routledge, 2013), 45–50; Ellen Beate Hansen Sandseter, interview with author, Trondheim, Norway, November 8, 2012; Elger Blitz, interview with author, November 14, 2012, Amsterdam, the Netherlands.

52. Dorothy Thornhill, mayor of Watford in Herdfordshire, e-mail to author, June 6, 2012.

53. Jane M. Healy, *Your Child's Growing Mind*, 3rd ed. (New York: Broadway Books, 2004), 31.

54. Chris Mercogliano, *In Defense of Childhood: Protecting Kids' Inner Wildness* (Boston: Beacon, 2007), 14–15.

55. Mintz, *Huck's Raft*, 340.

56. Ibid., 342.

57. Alexander Filip (deputy director of Office of Communications, CPSC), phone interview with author, August 15, 2013.

58. Wendy S. Grolnick, *The Psychology of Parental Control: How Well-Meant Parenting Backfires* (Mahwah, NJ: Lawrence Erlbaum Associates, 2003), 113–17. Grolnick cites relations theory, proposed by Alice Miller and Margaret Mahler in the 1980s, in which parents look to children to fill their own perceived deficits. She also notes Salvador Minuchin's

1970s work which found that all members of the family have become entwined without any hierarchical authority. She notes Stephen Sales's 1970s work showing that parents become more authoritarian when faced with a threat to their environment, while she also acknowledges that some of his work was disproved by Stanley and Karen Stenner in 1997.

59. Ashley E. Zielinski, Lynne M. Rochette, and Gary A. Smith, "Stair-Related Injuries to Young Children Treated in US Emergency Departments, 1999–2008," *Pediatrics* 129 (March 2012). The authors report almost 932,000 injuries over the nine-year period under study.

60. Wyver et al., "Ten Ways," 269.

61. Karl-Chirstian Thies, e-mail to author, July 24, 2012.

62. Centers for Disease Control and Prevention, "CDC Childhood Injury Report: Patterns of Unintentional Injuries among 0–19 Year Olds in the United States, 2000–2006" (2008)," cited in Mariana Brussoni, Lise L. Olsen, Ian Pike, and David A. Sleet, "Risky Play and Children's Safety: Balancing Priorities for Optimal Child Development," *International Journal of Environmental Research and Public Health* 9, no. 9 (September 2012): 3134–48.

63. Craig W. O'Brien, "Injuries and Investigated Death Associated with Play Equipment, 2001–2009." See cpsc.gov/pagefiles/108596/playground.pdf. According to O'Brien, only 1,574 incidents were actually reported to CPSC; this is different than the estimated hospital visits.

The U.S. Consumer Product Safety Commission issued a statement in 2001 that home playgrounds were the source of most fatalities between 1990 and 2001; most of these were caused by strangulation. The 2001 study was "Playground Equipment," available at www.cpsc.gov/CPSCPUB/PREREL/prhtm101/01213.html. It is worth noting that there were sixty deaths on public playgrounds during that decade; the number between 2001 and 2008 was forty. The attention to drawstrings on clothing has been slow but finally effective.

In February 1996, CPSC issued *guidelines about drawstrings* in children's upper outerwear. In 1997, those guidelines were incorporated into a voluntary standard (F-1816). There was a further letter urging action in May 2006 in which they reported a decline in fatalities compared with the period 1985 to 1997, when there had been at least twenty-one deaths from drawstrings. Letter from John Gibson Mullan, director, Office of Compliance, U.S. CPSC, to "manufacturers, Importers and Retailers of Children's Upper Outerwear." Then, in July 2011, based on the guidelines and voluntary standard, CPSC issued a federal regulation prohibiting drawstrings in outwear for the upper body of children.

64. Sandseter and Kennair, "Children's Risky Play," 275.

65. M. L. Waltzman et al., "Monkeybar Injuries: Complications of Play," *Pediatrics* 105, no. 5 (2000): 1174–75.

66. M. Paul Friedberg, interview with author, February 14, 2013, New York City.

67. John T. Gaffney, "Tibia Fractures in Children Sustained on a Playground Slide," *Journal of Pediatric Orthopedics* 29 (September 2009): 606–8. When Dr. John Gaffney, an orthopedist, looked at the number of tibia fractures that came to his office in an eleven-month period, he found fifty-eight. Only eight of those occurred on playgrounds, but all occurred when parents went down slides with children between fourteen and thirty-two months of age. His advice: "If the child is unable to use the slide independently, another activity would be more appropriate."

68. Lady Allen of Hurtwood, quoted in "Junkyard Playgrounds," *Time Magazine*, June 25, 1965, 71.

69. Jeremiah Clinton, "Playgrounds Home to Bumps, Bruises and Broken Bones," *Ravelli Republic*, April 2, 2013. Clinton, a Montana doctor who believes the benefits of playgrounds

outweigh any injuries, says that broken bones are part of growing up; he claims that 75 percent of boys and 50 percent of girls will fracture a limb before they become adults.

70. I am grateful to Robert Whitaker for pointing this out to me.

71. Nicholas Day, "Tear Down the Swing Sets," *Slate*, January 28, 2013.

72. For descriptions of Reform era playgrounds, see Galen Cranz, *The Politics of Park Design: A History of Urban Parks in America* (Cambridge: MIT Press, 1982; paperback ed., 1989), 62–87. See also Iannacone, "Neighborhood Playgrounds and Parks," 174.

73. Iannacone, "Neighborhood Playgrounds and Parks," 174.

74. Cecilia Perez and Roger A. Hart, "Beyond Playgrounds: Planning for Children's Access to the Environment," in *Innovation in Play Environments*, ed. Paul F. Wilkinson (New York: St. Martin's, 1980), 253. Perez and Hart, citing the Russell Sage Foundation report of 1914, say that the playgrounds were often empty while children looked for more interesting places.

75. Ibid., 144.

76. Ibid., 140.

77. Gary Cross, *Kids' Stuff: Toys and the Changing World of American Childhood* (Cambridge: Harvard University Press, 1997), 123.

78. For more information on this history, see Susan G. Solomon, *American Playgrounds: Revitalizing Community Space* (Hanover, NH: University Press of New England, 2005).

79. For a more detailed analysis and images, see ibid.

80. Donne Buck, e-mail to author, September 4, 2013.

81. Buck, e-mail to author, September 15, 2013. Buck also feels that the high tower may have led foreign visitors to believe that "the Adventure Playground meant large, overpowering climbing" and "that this erroneous conclusion damaged the physical development" in other countries.

82. Simon Nicholson, "How Not to Cheat Children: The Theory of Loose Parts," *Landscape Architecture* 62 (October 1971): 30–34.

83. Ibid.

84. Apted was actually a minor producer in the first filming; he came into his own in the second movie in the series, *14 Up.*

85. Paul F. Wilkinson and Robert S. Lockhart, "Safety in Children's Formal Play Environments," in Wilkinson, ed., *Innovation in Play Environments*, 85–96.

86. Wyver et al., "Ten Ways," 263. Tom Jambor devised the term "surplus safety"; the phenomenon is best seen, according to these authors, in Australia, the United Kingdom, and the United States.

87. Waller et al., "The Dynamics of Early Childhood Spaces," 440.

88. Ibid., 439.

89. Waller et al., "The Dynamics of Early Childhood Spaces," 438, 439–41.

90. Clause S. Fischer, *Made in America: A Social History of American Culture and Character* (Chicago: University of Chicago Press, 2010), 10.

91. Ibid., 242.

92. Fass, "The Child-Centered Family?" 16–17.

93. European Committee for Standardization (EN1176: 2008) "Playground Equipment and Surfacing—Part 1: General Safety Requirements and Test Method," quoted in Helen Little and David Eager, "Risk, Challenge, and Safety: Implications for Play Quality and Playground Design," *European Early Childhood Education Research Journal* 18, no. 4 (2010): 502.

94. CPSC, "Public Playground Safety Handbook," Introduction, November 2010.

95. Richard E. Nisbett has written a fascinating study of how Asian and Western thought are different that is very useful to this discussion. See Richard E. Nisbett, *The Geography of Thought: How Asians and Westerners Think Differently . . . and Why* (New York: Free Press, 2003). Nisbett also includes a reference to nineteenth-century German

social scientists, who made distinctions between collectivist and individualist societies; he prefers the terms "interdependent" and "independent" and cites Hazel Markus and Shinobu Kitayama as the scholars who coined those phrases (55–57). Nesbitt also recognizes that Americans, who tend to accept only one view at a time, avoid contradictions and seek rules to justify their choices. He maintains that Asian society, geared toward harmony, permits individuals to hold two contradictions at the same time in order to achieve compromise His analysis seems a brilliant appraisal of why Americans find it hard to understand nuances in our daily lives.

96. Hendry, *Understanding Japanese Society*, 45–50, 57, 223. Since the 1980s, Japan, where fewer than 30 percent of the married couples have children (2005), has attempted to underscore the role of the individual. See Peter Cave, *Primary School in Japan: Self, Individuality and Learning in Elementary Education* (New York: Routledge, 2007). Japan changed its school curriculum in 1998, with the changes going into effect in 2002. The new emphasis was on problem solving, learning to learn, creativity, and the integration of subjects. The consensus is that not a great deal has changed. I am grateful to Naomi Pollak, an American architect and architectural critic who has lived in Tokyo for many years, for her insights about how children navigate their way around the city. She pointed out that children do have buzzers on their backpacks if they need to signal someone nearby for help. Naomi Pollak, interview with author, May 27, 2013, Tokyo. Americans will, of course, see a vivid contrast with the way our society operates. In 2008, columnist Lenore Skenazy planned a route with her nine-year-old son so that he would be able to take the subway from a big department store to his Manhattan apartment, a journey of less than four miles. After writing about his successful trip, Skenazy was invited on news programs where the crawl

dubbed her "America's Worst Mom." She later reported that a poll on the website of one of the channels indicated that fewer than a third of the respondents endorsed what she had done. Lenore Skenazy, "More from America's Worst Mom," Huffington Post.com, April 4, 2008 (www.huffingtonpost.com/more-from -americas-worst-b-91675.html).

97. Chris Berthelsen (www.a-small-lab .com/), a New Zealander who has lived in Tokyo for more than a decade, has researched the city and children's roles in it. Berthelsen, telephone interview with author, June 9, 2013.

2. Risk and Independence

1. Susan Davis and Nancy Eppler-Wolff, *Raising Children Who Soar: A Guide to Healthy Risk-Taking in an Uncertain World* (New York: Teachers College Press, 2009), 15. A serious discussion about the value of risk began in the 1980s. For more insights into the notion of healthy risk taking, see Pia Christensen and Miguel Romero Mikkelsen, "Jumping Off and Being Careful: Children's Strategies of Risk Management in Everyday Life," *Sociology of Health and Illness* 30, no. 1 (2008): 112–30.

2. Helen Little and David Eager, "Risk, Challenge and Safety: Implications for Play Quality and Playground Design," *European Early Childhood Education Research Journal* 18, no. 4 (2010): 497–513.

3. Sandseter and Kennair, "Children's Risky Play," 257–84; Little and Eager, "Risk, Challenge and Safety," 497–513.

4. Mike Shooter and Sue Baily, eds. *The Young Mind* (London: Bantam Press and the Royal College of Psychiatrists, 2009), 47.

5. Lady Allen of Hurtwood, *Planning for Play* (London: Thames and Hudson, 1968). See also Betsy Thom, Rosemary Sales, and Jenny J. Pearce, "Introduction," in *Growing Up with Risk*, ed. Thom, Sales, and Pearce (Bristol: Policy, 2007). This book and other sources indicate that resilience, while discussed as a teachable attribute in the parenting literature, is usually

reserved for discussion of recovery from extreme events. Some scholars fear that the term "resiliency" has been diluted in parenting publications. See Diane M. Hoffman, "Risky Investments: Parenting and the Production of the 'Resilient Child,'" *Health, Risk and Society* 12 (August 2010): 385–94. Yet there is something engaging about the notion (Thom, Sales, and Pearce, eds., *Growing Up with Risk*, 1) that children's "capacity to draw on their own resources to withstand unpredictable events that are a part of everyday life is developed through taking risks and learning to cope with the unexpected." R. Gilligan, "Beyond Permanence? The Importance of Resilience in Child Placement Practices and Planning," *Adoption and Fostering* 21, no. 1 (1997): 12–20.

6. Ellen Beate Hansen Sandseter, "Categorizing Risky-Play: How Can We Identify Risk-Taking in Children's Play," *European Early Childhood Education Research Journal* 15, no. 2 (June 2007): 237–52.

7. Sandseter, "Characteristics of Risky Play," 4.

8. Sandseter and Kennair, "Children's Risky Play," 259.

9. Sandseter, "Categorizing Risky-Play," 238, 243.

10. Ibid., 248–49.

11. Ellen Beate Hansen Sandseter, "'It Tickles in My Tummy!': Understanding Children's Risk-taking in Play through Reversal Theory," *Journal of Early Childhood Research* 8, no. 1 (2010): 82–84.

12. Ellen Beate Hansen Sandseter, "Children's Expressions of Exhilaration and Fear in Risky Play," *Contemporary Issues in Early Childhood* 10, no. 2 (2009): 92–106.

13. Sandseter and Kennair, "Children's Risky Play," 257–84. The authors are very clear in noting that there have not been extensive deprivation studies on risk; in other words, we don't know for sure what happens when children do not encounter risk. Do they become more neurotic or fearful?

14. Aamodt and Wang, *Welcome to Your Child's Brain*, 129.

15. Ibid., 125.

16. Sandra Aamodt and Sam Wang, "Building Self-Control, the American Way," *New York Times*, February 17, 2012.

17. Christensen and Mikkelsen, "Jumping Off and Being Careful," 115.

18. Sandseter, "Categorizing Risky-Play," 238; Sandseter, "Children's Expressions of Exhilaration and Fear in Risky Play," 94.

19. Helen Little and Shirley Wyver, "Individual Difference in Children's Risk Perception and Appraisals in Outdoor Play Environments," *International Journal of Early Years Education* 18, no. 4 (December 2010): 297.

20. Sandseter, "Children's Expressions of Exhilaration and Fear in Risky Play," 101–2; Sandseter, "It Tickles in My Tummy!" 68. Sandseter cites Michael J. Apter's reversal theory (first developed in the 1980s).

21. Sandseter, "Children's Expressions of Exhilaration and Fear in Risky Play," 92–106.

22. Sandseter, "Characteristics of Risky Play," 8.

23. Richard Field acquired the tract of thirty acres in 1842. He set it up as an arboretum. Marquand acquired and enlarged the property in 1885. The park now has more than two hundred specimen trees and several paths. A private foundation for the enhancement of the park was created in 1953 at the time the park was established and still helps Princeton with maintenance.

24. The obituary for Elinor Forseyth, January 12, 1983, *Town Topics* newspaper, indicates that she designed the sand pit after being inspired by a trip to Japan.

25. Sandseter and Kennair, "Children's Risky Play," 258, 260, 261.

26. Patty Donald (founding director), interview with author, February 27, 2013, Berkeley, CA.

27. Sandseter, "Characteristics of Risky Play," 14.

28. Ellen Beate Hansen Sandseter, Helen Little and Shirley Wyver, "Do Theory and Pedagogy Have an Impact on Provision for Outdoor Learning? A Comparison of Australia and Norway," *Journal of Adventure Education and Outdoor Learning* 12, no. 3 (2012): 167–70; Wenche Aasen, Liv Torunn Grindheim, and Jane Waters, "The Outdoor Environment as a Site for Children's Participation, Meaning-Making and Democratic Learning: Examples from Norwegian Kindergartens," *International Journal of Primary, Elementary and Early Years Education* 37 (2009): 6.

29. Wyver et al., "Ten Ways," 267.

30. Aasen et al., "The Outdoor Environment," 8.

31. Sandseter, interview with author, November 8, 2012.

32. See "Emerging Architects," *Architectural Review* 230 (December 2011): 62; Dan Zohar, telephone conversation with author, June 29, 2012.

33. "Emerging Architects," 62.

34. Trondheim Master Plan 2001–12, quoted in Per Christiansen, *Kunst ute, Kunst inne: Utsmykking Trondheim/Public Art in Trondheim 2000–2010* (Trondheim: Taour Akademisk Forlag, 2010), 13. In the case of public-private partnership, the two entities split the cost of the artwork.

35. Atsushi Kitagawara, answers to e-mail questions, translated by Kathrin Sauerwein, e-mail to author, June 24, 2013.

36. Ibid.

37. Information on this project comes from Clément Willemin, telephone conversation (June 29, 2012) and interview (November 26, 2012) with the author, Paris.

38. Willemin, interview with author, November 26, 2012.

39. Ibid.

40. Sandseter, "Characteristics of Risky Play," 5–9.

41. Liane Lefairve and Henk Döll, *Ground-Up City: Play as a Design Tool* (Rotterdam: Nai 010, 2007).

42. Elger Blitz, interview with author, November 12 and 14, 2012, Amsterdam.

43. Information on this project comes from the press information kit prepared by the Copenhagen office of Bjarke Ingles Group (BIG).

44. "Playing Merry Games on Waldorf Roof," *New York Times*, March 30, 1909. Apparatus included swings and "swinging rings."

45. Sandseter and Kennair, "Children's Risky Play," 259.

46. Helen Little, Shirley Wyver, and Frances Gibson, "The Influence of Play Context and Adult Attitudes on Young Children's Physical Risk-Taking during Outdoor Play," *European Early Childhood Education Research Journal* 19, no. 1 (2011): 128.

47. Henry Jenkins, cited in Steven Mintz, "The Changing Face of Children's Culture," in Fass and Grossberg, eds., *Reinventing Childhood after World War II*, 49.

48. Jane McGonigal, *Reality Is Broken: Why Games Make Us Better and How They Can Change the World* (New York: Penguin, 2011), 3.

49. Ibid., 28, 31–33.

50. Ibid., 21–29. She discusses flow on pages 35 to 40. Mihály Csíkszentmihályi first defined flow in the 1970s. There is no universal agreement on whether young children can actually experience flow.

51. Eriksen, *Playground Design*, 3.

3. Failing and Succeeding

1. Little, Wyver, and Gibson, "The Influence of Play Context," 127.

2. Sandseter, "Children's Expressions of Exhilaration and Fear in Risky Play," 103.

3. Sandseter, "It Tickles in My Tummy!" 78.

4. Grolnick, *The Psychology of Parental Control*, 1–19.

5. Madeline Levine, *The Price of Privilege* (New York: Harper Collins, 2006), 79.

6. Kristina R. Olson and Carol S. Dweck, "Social Cognitive Development: A New Look," *Child Development Perspectives* 3, no. 1 (2009):

60. Dweck summarizes her findings for a general audience in her book *Mindset: The New Psychology of Success* (New York: Random House, 2006).

7. Adele Diamond, "The Evidence Base for Improving School Outcomes by Addressing the Whole Child and by Addressing Skills and Attitudes, Not Just Content," *Early Education and Development* 21, no. 5 (2010): 786.

8. Ibid.

9. Perez and Hart, "Beyond Playgrounds," 254.

10. Todd Rader and Amy Crews, interview with author, September 10, 2012, Brooklyn, New York.

11. Paul Andreas and Peter Cachola Schmal, *Takaharu + Yui Tezuka: Nostalgic Future* [catalog for exhibition] (Frankfurt am Main: Deutsches Architeckturmuseum DAM, 2009), 32–47. Additional information on this project comes from architects Takaharu Tezuka and Yui Tezuka, interview with author, May 28, 2013, Tokyo; Sekiichi Kato, principal of Fuji Montessori School, and Sara Tabata, translator and aide at Fuji Montessori School, interview with author, May 23, 2013, Tokyo.

12. Taro Igarashi, "'Straight Modern,' or the Intensity of Architecture," in ibid., 12.

13. Toshiko Horiuchi MacAdam and Charles MacAdam, telephone interview with author, March 25, 2013; Takaharu Tezuka and Yui Tezuka, interview with author, May 23, 2013, Tokyo.

14. Mark Christensen, city manager of Saratoga Springs, Utah, telephone conversation with author, May 9, 2012.

15. Held in conjunction with MoMA's exhibition *Century of the Child*, the symposium took place October 19, 2012.

16. Isolde Raftery, "Park Domes Fenced Off to Protect Children," *New York Times*, June 18, 2010. A follow-up piece appeared as "The Domes Are Gone," *New York Times*, June 29, 2010.

17. Monica Adams, interview with author,

November 13, 2012, Rotterdam; and e-mail from Adams to author, January 28, 2013.

18. Helle Nebelong, interview with author, December 12, 2011, Copenhagen.

19. Helle Nebelong, quoted in Susan G. Solomon, "Artful Playscapes," *Public Art Review*, no. 45 (Fall/Winter 2011): 50.

20. Elger Blitz, interview with author, November 12 and November 14, 2012, Amsterdam.

21. Roger Hart, "Containing Children: Some Lessons on Planning for Play from New York City," *Environment and Urbanization* 14 (2002): 135–48.

22. Wyver et al., "Ten Ways," 264.

23. Karen E. Adolph, "Learning to Move," *Current Directions in Psychological Science* 17, no 3 (2008): 217.

24. Healy, *Your Child's Growing Mind*, 93.

4. Executive Function

1. Charlie Lewis and Jeremy I. M. Carpendale, "Introduction to 'Social Interaction and the Development of Executive Function,'" a special issue of *New Direction for Child and Adolescent Development* 123 (Spring 2009): 2–3. Lewis and Carpendale illustrate the differing definitions of EF. They believe that sequencing and planning are secondary aspects of EF that are necessary skills for working memory to be efficient.

2. Diamond, "The Evidence Base for Improving School Outcomes," 782.

3. Adele Diamond and Kathleen Lee, "Interventions Shown to Aid Executive Function Development in Children 4 to 12 Years Old," *Science Magazine* 333, no. 6045 (August 19, 2011): 959.

4. Ibid. See also the work of T. E. Moffitt on childhood self-control as summarized in Adele Diamond, "Activities and Programs That Improve Children's Executive Functions," *Current Directions in Psychological Science* 21 (2012): 335–41.

5. Adele Diamond et al., "Preschool Program Improves Cognitive Control," *Science* 318, no. 5855 (November 30, 2007): 1387–88. Because poor kids have disproportionately low EF skills, they sometimes never catch up in school.

6. Brittany L. Rhoades et al., "Demographic and Familial Predictors of Early Executive Function Development: Contribution of a Person-Centered Perspective," *Journal of Experimental Child Psychology* 108 (March 2011): 638–62.

The concept of "emotional intelligence" is still debated. Peter Salovey and John D. Mayer, who first defined it in 1990, believe that the concept has been hijacked by popular interpretations, such as those by Daniel Goleman, that have overstated what it is and how it can be applied. See Peter Salovey, Marc A. Brackett, and John D. Mayer, *Emotional Intelligence: Key Reading on the Mayer and Salovey Model* (Port Chester, NY: Dude, 2004).

7. Susan H. Landry, Karen E. Smith, and Paul R. Swank, "New Directions in Evaluating Social Problem Solving in Childhood: Early Precursors and Links to Adolescent Social Competence," *New Directions for Child and Adolescent Development* 123 (Spring 2009): 51–68.

8. Angel L. Duckworth and Martin E. P. Seligman, "Self-Discipline Outdoes IQ in Predicting Academic Performance of Adolescents," *Psychological Science* 16 (December 2005): 939–44.

9. Walter Mischel, Yuichi Shoda, and Philip K. Peake, "The Nature of Adolescent Competencies Predicted by Preschool Delay of Gratification," *Journal of Personality and Social Psychology* 54, no. 4 (1988): 687–96. Among the most important follow-up studies are Inge-Marie Eigsti et al., "Predicting Cognitive Control from Preschool to Late Adolescence and Young Adulthood," *Psychological Science* 17, no. 6 (2006): 478–84; Gopnik, *The Philosophical Baby*, 58–60. Gopnik, who works on issues of cognitive development, critiqued Mischel's old experiments, characterizing them as mean-spirited, since children need to be somewhere

between three and five to exercise real self-control. She notes that the successful children could resist temptations by fantasizing about the objects and thinking they were something less tempting than a delicious snack.

10. Sue Robson, "Self-regulation and Metacognition in Young Children's Self-initiated Play and Reflective Dialogue," *International Journal of Early Years Education* 18, no. 3 (September 2010): 227–41, 228.

11. Paul Tough, *How Children Succeed: Grit, Curiosity, and the Hidden Power of Character* (Boston: Houghton Mifflin, 2012), 21.

12. Medina, *Brain Rules for Baby*.

13. Aamodt and Wang, *Welcome to Your Child's Brain*, 115–16.

14. Dan Zohar, telephone interview with author, November 8, 2012.

15. Christiansen, *Kunst ute, Kunst inne*, 62–63.

16. Thomas Moser and Marianne T. Martinsen, "The Outdoor Environment in Norwegian Kindergartens as Pedagogical Space for Toddlers' Play, Learning and Development," *European Early Childhood Education Research Journal* 18, no. 4 (2010): 462.

17. Rob Gregory and Catherine Slessor, "Fireplace for Children," *Architectural Review* 226 (December 2009): 102–3.

18. Peter Walker, interview with author, February 27, 2013; David Walker, interview with author, November 1, 2012, Berkeley, CA.

19. Diamond and Lee, "Interventions Shown to Aid Executive Function Development," 959.

20. John R. Best, Patricia H. Miller, and Lara L. Jones, "Executive Functions after Age 5: Changes and Correlates," *Developmental Review* 29 (2009): 187–88.

21. Diamond, "Activities and Programs," 336.

22. Alex Gilliam (founder of Public Workshop), telephone interview with author, August 23, 2013.

23. Staempfli, "Reintroducing Adventure," 270; Dorothee Jahn, "Adventures Abound," *Tokyo Weekender*, May 20, 2010. Staemfpli says that there are a thousand adventure

playgrounds spread among the United Kingdom, Denmark, and Germany. Jahn refers to two hundred adventure playgrounds in Japan, a number that reappears in other listings. Handout information from the Japan Adventure Playground Association indicates that the number of active adventure playgrounds is much smaller — especially the number that are permanent. I am grateful to Masako Irie, Shuto Machko, Michiko Ono Paddock, and Riho Tanaka for their hospitality and information at the Henegi and Toyama adventure playgrounds in Tokyo.

24. Masako Irie (a founding parent of Toyama Playpark), interview with author, May 27, 2013, Tokyo.

25. Diamond, "The Evidence Base for Improving School Outcomes," 783–84.

26. Play worker Penny Wilson to author, e-mail, July 11, 2013.

27. Joe L. Frost and Barry L. Klein, *Children's Play and Playgrounds* (Boston: Allyn and Bacon, 1979), 132–41.

28. Play worker Marcus Schmidt, e-mail communication with author, October 3, 2012.

29. Information on this project comes from Marc Hacker, interview with author, March 21, 2012, New York City; Nancy Barthold, interview with author, March 21, 2013, New York City; phone conversation with Adrian Benepe, October 11, 2013.

30. "Play ranger" is another term used for play worker. They are also described as "unobtrusive guides," "play mediator," or "play shaman," as cited in Staempfli, "Reintroducing Adventure," 271.

31. Diamond et al., "Preschool Program Improves Cognitive Control," 1387.

32. Dimitri Christakis, Frederick J. Zimmerman, and Michelle M. Garrison, "Effect of Block Play on Language Acquisition and Attention in Toddlers," *Archives of Pediatrics and Adolescent Medicine* 161, no. 10 (2007): 968.

33. Day, "Tear Down the Swing Sets."

34. Ken Smith, interview with author,

February 7, 2013, New York City; Peter Reed, *Groundswell: Constructing the Contemporary Landscape* (New York: Museum of Modern Art, 2005), 80–83.

35. Lina Engelen et al., "Increasing Physical Activity in Young Primary School Children— It's Child's Play: A Cluster Randomised Trial," *Preventive Medicine* 56 (2013): 319–20.

36. Anita Bundy et al., "The Risk Is That There Is 'No Risk': A Simple, Innovative Intervention to Increase Children's Activity Levels," *International Journal of Early Years Education* 17, no. 1 (March 2009): 33–45.

37. Diamond, "Activities and Programs," 336.

38. Diamond, "Strategies and Programs That Help to Improve Executive Functions in Young Children," presentation at the American Psychological Association, August 2009, Toronto Canada; Diamond and Lee, "Interventions Shown to Aid Executive Function Development," 961.

39. Bodrova and Leong, *Tools of the Mind*, 35.

40. Gopnik, *The Philosophical Baby*, 37.

41. Po Bronson and Ashley Merryman, *Nurture Shock: New Thinking about Children* (New York: Twelve, 2009), 171, 173.

42. Cynthia L. Elias and Laura E. Berk, "Self-regulation in Young Children: Is There a Role for Socio-dramatic Play?" *Early Childhood Research Quarterly* 17 (2002): 218–19.

43. Dunn, *Children's Friendships*, 28.

44. Paul L. Harris, *The Work of the Imagination* (Malden, MA: Blackwell, 2000), 47.

45. Todd Rader and Amy Crews, interview with author, September 10, 2012, Brooklyn, New York.

46. Adele Diamond, "The Interplay of Biology and the Environment Broadly Defined," *Developmental Psychology* 45 (2009): 4.

47. Charles H. Hillman, Kirk I. Erickson, and Arthur F. Kramer, "Be Smart, Exercise Your Heart: Exercise Effects on Brain and Cognition," *Nature* 9 (January 2008): 58–65.

48. Sarah Munro et al., "Dramatically Larger Flanker Effects," presentation at the annual meeting of the Cognitive Neuroscience Society, San Francisco, CA, April 9, 2006).

49. Diamond and Lee, "Interventions Shown to Aid Executive Function Development," 959–64.

50. Diamond, "Activities and Programs," 337.

51. Diamond and Lee, "Interventions Shown to Aid Executive Function Development," 961.

52. Laura Chaddock et al., "Role of Childhood Aerobic Fitness in Successful Street Crossing," *Medicine and Science in Sports and Exercises* (2012): 750. Some of the same authors—Chaddock, Hillman, and Kramer; see ibid.—participated with other authors in a companion study, "A Functional MRI Investigation of the Association between Childhood Aerobic Fitness and Neurocognitive Control," *Biological Psychology* 89 (2012): 260–68. With a different set of colleagues they published "Childhood Aerobic Fitness Predicts Cognitive Performance One Year Later," *Journal of Sports Sciences* 30, no. 5 (March 2012): 421–30.

53. Chaddock et al., "Role of Childhood Aerobic Fitness," 752–53.

54. Diamond, "The Interplay of Biology," 4.

55. Diamond, "The Evidence Base for Improving School Outcomes," 784.

56. "Physical Activity Guidelines for Americans" (2008), www.health.gov /PAGuidelines/pdf/PAguide.pdf. This is less demanding than the guidelines of the National Association for Sport and Physical Education, which suggests cumulative times of thirty minutes a day of structured physical activity and sixty minutes a day of unstructured physical activity for toddlers; and sixty minutes of structured activity then sixty minutes a day of vigorous physical activity (at least several should be more than fifteen minutes long) for preschoolers. They suggest at least sixty minutes of activity on most days for children five to twelve. See www.aahperd.org/naspe /standards/nationalGuidelines/ActiveStart.cfm. Interestingly, the Canadian guidelines suggest that children under five get 180

minutes of physical activity, of any kind, until they reach five, at which point that activity can be reduced to 60 minutes. Line Tremblay, Celine Boudreau-Larivière, and Krystel Cimon-Lambert, "Promoting Physical Activity in Preschoolers: A Review of the Guidelines, Barriers, and Facilitators for Implementation of Policies and Practices," *Canadian Psychology* 53, no. 4 (November 2012): 280–90.

57. Kirsten K. Davison and Catherine T. Lawson, "Do Attributes in the Physical Environment Influence Children's Physical Activity? A Review of the Literature," *International Journal of Behavioral Nutrition and Physical Activity* 3 (2006), available at www.ijbnpa.org/content/3/1/19.

58. Yovanka B. Lobo and Adam Winsler, "The Effects of a Creative Dance and Movement Program on the Social Competence of Head Start Preschoolers," *Social Development* 15 (2006): 501–19.

59. Diamond and Lee, "Interventions Shown to Aid Executive Function Development," 961.

5. Friendship

1. Dunn, *Children's Friendships*, 7, 29, 156–57.

2. Diamond and Lee, "Interventions Shown to Aid Executive Function Development," 961.

3. Emily Bazelon, "American Kids Don't Know How to Explore. Maybe What They Need Is Forest Kindergarten," *Slate*, December 4, 2013.

4. Zigler and Bishop-Josef, "The Cognitive Child versus the Whole Child," 19. While these authors maintain that respect for play declined after the launch of Sputnik, this idea is negated by the expansion of interesting playgrounds until the 1970s.

5. Anthony D. Pellegrini, *Recess: Its Role in Education and Development* (Mahwah, NJ: Lawrence Erlbaum Associates, 2005), 5.

6. Smith, *Children and Play*, 201–4.

7. Pellegrini, *Recess*, 153.

8. Smith, *Children and Play*, 118–19, 202; D. J. Bjorlund and B. L. Green, "Adaptive Nature of

Cognitive Immaturity," *American Psychologist* 47 (1992): 46–54.

9. Sara Bennett and Nancy Kalish, *The Case against Homework: How Homework Is Hurting Our Children and What We Can Do About It* (New York: Crown Publishers, 2006). This is one of several recent assessments on the worthlessness of homework, especially in the lower grades. The authors quote Etta Kralovec, who cowrote (with John Buell) *The End of Homework: How Homework Disrupts Families, Overburdens Children, and Limits Learning*, Boston: Beacon Press, 2000. Kralovec, cited on page 13, write that "There's been no research done on whether homework teaches responsibility, self-discipline, or motivation."

10. Robert Murray and Catherine Ramstetter, for the Council on School Health of the American Academy of Pediatrics, "Policy Statement: The Crucial Role of Recess in School," *Pediatrics* 131, no. 1 (January 2013): 183–88.

11. Anthony D. Pellegrini and Robyn M. Holmes, "The Role of Recess in Primary School," in Singer, Golinkoff, and Hirsh-Pasek, eds., *Play = Learning*, 50.

12. Anthony D. Pellegrini and Catherine M. Bohn, "The Role of Recess in Children's Cognitive Performance and School Adjustment," *Educational Researcher* 34, no. 1 (January/February 2005): 14.

13. Pellegrini and Holmes, "The Role of Recess in Primary School," 50–51.

14. Pellegrini, "Rough-and-Tumble Play," 112.

15. Sandseter and Kennair, "Children's Risky Play," 265–72.

16. Anthony D. Pellegrini, "Elementary School Children's Rough-and-Tumble Play," *Early Childhood Research Quarterly* 4 (1989): 245–60.

17. Richard Fletcher, Jennifer StGeorge, and Emily Freeman, "Rough and Tumble Play Quality: Theoretical Foundation for a New Measure of Father-Child Interaction," *Early*

Child Development and Care 183, no. 6 (June 2012): 746.

18. Jaak Panksepp, quoted in Steven Johnson, *Mind Wide Open: Your Brain and the Neuroscience of Everyday Life* (New York: Scribner, 2005), 126.

19. McGonigal, *Reality Is Broken*, 84.

20. Smith, *Children and Play*, 111.

21. T. L. Reed and M. Brown, "The Expression of Care in the Rough and Tumble Play of Boys," *Journal of Research in Childhood Education* 15, no. 1: 104–16; Pellegrini, *The Role of Play in Human Development*, 10, 98. Pellegrini shows that the idea of a positive "play face" has been discussed since the 1970s.

22. Reed and Brown, "The Expression of Care in the Rough and Tumble Play of Boys," 113.

23. Bundy et al., "The Risk Is That There Is 'No Risk,'" 33–45.

24. Cary J. Roseth et al., "Teacher Intervention and U.S. Preschoolers' Natural Conflict Resolution after Aggressive Competition," *Behaviour* 145 (2008): 1620.

25. Kilvington and Wood, *Reflective Playwork*, 77.

26. Anthony D. Pellegrini, "Rough-and-Tumble Play from Childhood through Adolescence: Development and Possible Functions," in *Blackwell Handbook of Childhood Social Development*, ed. Peter K. Smith and Craig H. Hart (Malden, MA: Wiley-Blackwell, 2004), 439.

27. Pellegrini, "Rough-and-Tumble Play," 112.

28. Ibid., 440.

29. Information on this project comes from Césare Peeren, interview with author, November 13, 2012, Rotterdam; Sabine van Dijk (instructor at Kinderparadijs Meidoorn), phone interview with author, June 11, 2013, and e-mail to author, June 24, 2013. While the local governmental ward has been providing funding, a city reorganization means that Kinderparadijs will have to apply to the city for funding in 2014.

30. Pellegrini and Bohn, "The Role of Recess," 13.

31. Huiyoung Shin and Allison M. Ryan, "How Do Adolescents Cope with Social Problems: An Examination of Social Goals, Coping with Friends, and Social Adjustment," *Journal of Early Adolescence* 32, no. 6 (2012): 852.

32. Lefaivre, *Ground-Up City*, 58–59.

33. Joy Hendry, e-mail to author, February 18, 2013.

34. Gamze Abramov and Yossi Abramov, telephone conversation with author, June 26, 2012; Nicky Washida, e-mail to author, June 19, 2012. Gamze Abramov and Nicky Washida are Westerners who lived in Japan for several years when they each had small children.

35. Washida, e-mail.

36. Robert Aspinall, e-mail to author, January 8, 2013.

37. Washida, e-mail.

38. Shelia M. Kennison and Elisabeth Ponce-Garcia, "The Role of Childhood Relationships with Older Adults in Reducing Risk-Taking by Young Adults," *Journal of Intergenerational Relationships* 10 (2012): 22–23. The authors see their conclusions as a validation of "terror management theory."

39. Ibid., 22.

40. Information about this project comes from Avi Laiser, telephone conversation with author, July 21, 2012.

41. Kalevi Korpela, Marketta Kyttä, and Terry Hartig, "Restorative Experience, Self-Regulation, and Children's Place Preferences," *Journal of Environmental Psychology* 22 (2002): 388, 389, 395.

42. Information on this project comes from Clément Willemin, interview with author, November 26, 2012, Paris, and e-mail to author, June 24, 2013.

43. Clement Willemin, e-mail to author, June 24, 2013.

44. Reinhard Kropf, principal of Helen & Hard, telephone interview with author, August 11, 2011.

45. Information on this project comes from Maki Onishi, e-mail to author, June 28, 2013. T Point, a Japanese business, was a major supporter of this project.

6. Nature and Exploration

1. One example is the RFP that the Portland, Oregon, Parks and Recreation Department issued in October 2011. They sought proposals for a "nature-based creative play area" in Westmoreland Park. The city hoped that this would be a pilot project for turning other parks into nature zones.

2. Liz O'Brien, "Learning Outdoors: The Forest School Approach," *Education 3–13: International Journal of Primary, Elementary and Early Years Education* 37 (February 2009): 45–46.

3. Jane Waters and Sharon Begley, "Supporting the Development of Risk Taking Behaviours in the Early Years: An Exploratory Study," *International Journal of Primary, Elementary and Early Years Education* 35, no. 4 (May 2008): 368.

4. Tim Gill, as quoted in Susan G. Solomon, "Artful Playscapes," *Public Art Review*, no. 45 (Fall/Winter 2011): 50.

5. Diane Steinle, "New Dunedin Playground Recalls Naturalist's Love of the Outdoors," *Tampa Bay Times*, August 2, 2013.

6. See www.polkcountyiowa.gov /conservation/things-to-do/jester-park-natural -playscape/.

7. Laila Niklasson and Anette Sandberg, "Children and the Outdoor Environment," *European Early Childhood Education Research Journal* 18, no. 4 (2010): 487.

8. "Is Contact with Nature Important for Healthy Child Development: State of the Evidence," in *Children and Their Environments: Learning, Using and Designing Spaces*, ed. Christopher Spencer and Mark Blades (Cambridge: Cambridge University Press, 2006), 136.

9. Andrea Faber Taylor and Frances E. (Ming) Kuo, "Could Exposure to Everyday Green Spaces Help Treat ADHD? Evidence from Children's Play Settings," *Applied Psychology: Health and Well-Being* 3 (2011): 284.

10. Rachel Hine, Jules Pretty, and Jo Barton, *Research Project: Social, Psychological and Cultural Benefits of Large Natural Habitat & Wilderness Experience: A Review of Current Literature for the Wilderness Foundation* (Colchester: University of Essex, 2009), 26.

11. Stephen R. Kellert, "Experiencing Nature: Affective, Cognitive, and Evaluative Development in Children," in *Children and Nature: Psychological, Sociocultural, and Evolutionary Investigations*, ed. Peter H. Kahn, Jr., and Stephen R. Kellert (Cambridge: MIT Press, 2002), 139.

12. See, for instance, the inspirational story in Robin C. Moore and Herbert H. Wong, *Natural Learning: The Life History of an Environmental Schoolyard* (Berkeley, CA: MIG Communications, 1997). For more information, see Solomon, *American Playgrounds*, 72–75.

13. Moore and Wong, *Natural Learning*.

14. Wyver et al., "Ten Ways," 267.

15. Ellen Beate Hansen Sandseter, "Restrictive Safety or Unsafe Freedom? Norwegian ECEC Practitioners' Perceptions and Practices Concerning Children's Risky Play," *Child Care in Practice* 18 (2012): 87.

16. Ibid., 276.

17. Ibid., 83–101 (quotations on 90, 87).

18. Ellen Beate Hansen Sandseter, e-mail to author, May 6, 2013.

19. Elger Blitz, interview with author, November 14, 2012, Amsterdam.

20. Robert Cervero and Cathleen Sullivan, "Kid-Friendly TODs," working paper, Institute of Urban and Regional Development, University of California, Berkeley, August 2010.

21. Andrea Broaddus, "Tale of Two Ecosuburbs in Freiburg, Germany: Encouraging Transit and Bicycle Use by Restricting Parking Provision," *Transportation Research Record* 2187 (2010): 114–22.

22. Helle Nebelong, interview with author, December 11, 2011, Copenhagen.

23. Diamond, "The Evidence Base for Improving School Outcomes," 785–86.

24. Nebelong, interview with author, December 12, 2011; and e-mail to author, February 17, 2013.

25. Pål Bøyesen, e-mail to author, June 25, 2013. I owe special thanks to Bøyesen, who works at the adjacent ReMida recycling facility, for answering my questions and locating a picture of the schoolyard when the school was on summer break.

26. Matthew Urbanski, principal of Michael van Valkenburgh Associates, interview with author, June 6, 2013, Brooklyn, NY.

27. Information for this project comes from a phone conversation with Patrick Dougherty, July 16, 2013; and an interview with Karyn Flynn (CEO and executive director) and staff — Rose Kelly and Scott Dahlman — of the Bay Area Discovery Museum, October 22, 2013.

28. Information for this project comes from e-mail correspondence between Randi Augenstein of HHA and author, August 22, 2013.

7. Paths

1. Whitney North Seymour, Jr., ed., *Small Urban Spaces: The Philosophy, Design, Sociology, and Politics of Vest-Pocket Parks and Other Small Urban Open Spaces* (New York: New York University Press, 1969).

2. Jennifer Isacoff, director of Parks for People, Bay Area program, phone conversation, October 21, 2013.

3. Roger Hart, panel participant at Municipal Art Society discussion, January 31, 2006; telephone conversation with author, April 22, 2013.

4. Yashar Hanstad, interview with author, November 7, 2012, Trondheim.

5. Interview with Andreas G. Gjertsen, *Floornature*, June 5, 2012, available at www.floornature.com/architects/interview/andreas-g-gjertsen-t.

6. Sarah Williams Goldhagen, "The Revolution at Your Community Library: New Media, New Community Centers," *New Republic*, March 9, 2013.

7. David Owen, "The Psychology of Space: Can a Norwegian Firm Solve the Problems of Times Square?" *New Yorker*, January 21, 2013. For information on Casa da Musica skateboard program, see http://bip.inescporto.pt/en/96/noticia07.html.

8. Mike Lanza, *Playborhood: Turn Your Neighborhood into a Place for Play* (Menlo Park, CA: Free Play, 2012).

9. Matthew Urbanski, principal of Michael van Valkenburgh Associates, interview with author, June 10, 2013, Brooklyn, New York.

10. Teri Hendy, phone interview with author, May 3, 2013.

11. Bundy et al., "The Risk Is That There Is 'No Risk,'" 35.

12. Tim Gill, *No Fear: Growing Up in a Risk-Averse Society* (London: Calouste Gulbenkian Foundation, 2007), 37–38. Gill has been a terrific ally, and I thank him for helping me understand the changing philosophy and players who altered risk-benefit analysis in England.

13. Robin Sutcliffe (chair of the Play Safety Forum) and Adrian Voce (then director of Play England), foreword, *Managing Risk in Play Provision: Implementation Guide* (2002, and expanded by Play England, 2008), 5. Published by the National Children's Bureau, this document was updated in 2012.

14. Ibid. Sutcliffe and Voce allude to "Staying Safe: The Government's Safeguarding Strategy," DCSF 2008b. Sutcliffe and Voce note that this document has had an impact on the revised European standards and the creation of a European Play Safety Forum.

15. Tim Gill, e-mail to author, October 17, 2013.

16. Little and Eager, "Risk, Challenge and Safety," 501.

17. Ibid., 106.

18. Barbara Kaucky, principal of erect architecture, phone conversation with author, October 22, 2013.

19. Natalie Canning, "The Influence of the Outdoor Environment: Den-Making in Three Contexts," *European Early Childhood Education Research Journal* 8, no. 4 (2010): 557.

20. Sara Knight, *Risk and Adventure in Early Years Outdoor Play: Learning from Forest Schools* (London: Sage Publications, 2011), 5.

21. David Montgomery, "Creating the Park of the Future," *Washington Post*, September 13, 2013.

22. Office of the Mayor, City of Chicago, press release, March 14, 2013.

23. John Byrne, "Emanuel Moves Playgrounds to Front of Park District Line," *Chicago Tribune*, March 14, 2013. Byrne's report of Emanuel's announcement is more specific than the press release. Community and neighborhood organizations applied for playground renovation funds through the city's wards.

24. Adrian Benepe, director of City Park Development, phone conversation with author, October 11, 2013; and Jennifer Isacoff, director of Parks for People in the Bay Area, October 21, 2013. TPL commissioned a report from the Rand Corporation in which Deborah Cohen, Terry Marsh, and others assessed the way Fitness Zones have affected neighborhoods in Los Angeles. The investigators found that usership increased, especially among people for whom parks were not a usual venue and who improved their activity from moderate to vigorous.

Conclusion: Paradigms

1. Blaine Merker, "Taking Place: Rebar's Absurd Tactics in Generous Urbanism," in *Insurgent Public Space: Guerrilla Urbanism and the Remaking of Contemporary Cities*, ed. Jeffrey Hou (New York: Routledge, 2010), 49.

2. John King, "SF Parklets a Homegrown Effort," *San Francisco Chronicle*, July 9, 2012; Matt Passmore, interview with author, Berkeley, CA, December 21, 2012. See also Merker, "Taking Place," 45.

3. Josh Stephens, "Parklets Create Public Space, 120 Square Feet at a Time," *California Planning and Development Report*, June 28, 2011, available at www.cp-dr.com/node/2977. Stephens says that the initial costs are approximately $1,000 for fees, $650 to remove two parking meters, plus construction. Each sponsor has to maintain $1 million of liability insurance.

4. Audi sponsored this space, but their commercial involvement seems to be limited to a discreet sign or each side of the street.

5. Information on this project comes from an interview with Elger Blitz of Carve, November 14, 2012, Amsterdam.

6. M. Paul Friedberg, interview with author, February 14, 2013, New York City.

7. Jackie Safier, interview with author, February 25, 2013; Meredith Thomas, interview with author, February 25, 2013; Nancy Madynski, interview with author, February 26, 2013; all in San Francisco.

8. Steven Koch, telephone interview with author, January 16, 2013.

9. Steven Koch, telephone interview with author, January 16, 2013. Columbia Cascade, a commercial manufacturer, was able to carry out most of the custom work.

10. Information on this project comes from Javier Malo de Molina (Burgos & Garrido Arquitectos), telephone interview with author, June 13, 2013, and discussion with author, November 18, 2013, Madrid and Peter Heuken (Richter), telephone interview with author, June 4, 2013.

11. Paige Johnson, founder of Playscapes blog, email to author, January 15, 2014.

12. *Alfred Ledermann and Alfred Trachsel, Creative Playgrounds and Recreation Centers* (New York: Frederick A. Praeger, 1959, 1968).

13. Lady Allen of Hurtwood, *Planning for Play* (London: Thames and Hudson, 1968), 15.

14. Ibid., 18.

15. Ibid.

16. Ibid., 16.

17. Ibid., 15.

18. Ibid., 20.

19. Ibid., 17.

20. Whitaker, phone interview with author, February 26, 2013.

21. Robert Whitaker, telephone interview with author, February 26, 2013.

Selected Bibliography

Aamodt, Sandra, and Sam Wang. *Welcome to Your Child's Brain*. New York: Bloomsbury, 2011.

Aasen, Wenche, Liv Torunn Grindheim, and Jane Waters. "The Outdoor Environment as a Site for Children's Participation, Meaning-making and Democratic Learning: Examples from Norwegian Kindergartens." *International Journal of Primary, Elementary and Early Years Education* 37 (2009): 5–13.

Adolph, Karen E. "Learning to Move." *Current Directions in Psychological Science* 17, no. 3 (2008): 213–18.

Allen, Lady, of Hurtwood. *Planning for Play*. London: Thames and Hudson, 1968.

Andreas, Paul, and Peter Cachola Schmal. *Takaharu + Yui Tezuka: Nostalgic Future*. Frankfurt am Main: Deutsches Architeckturmuseum DAM, 2009.

Andreasen, Nancy C. *The Creative Brain: The Science of Genius*. London: Plume, 2006 (originally published as *The Creating Brain: The Neuroscience of Genius*, 2005).

Ball, David J. "Ships in the Night and the Quest for Safety." *Injury Control and Safety Promotion* 7, no. 2 (2000): 83–96.

———. "Policy Issues and Risk-benefit Trade Offs of 'Safer Surfacing' for Children's Playgrounds." *Accident Analysis and Prevention* 36, no. 4 (July 2004): 661–70.

———. "Trends in Fall Injuries Associated with Children's Outdoor Climbing Frames." *International Journal of Injury Control and Safety Promotion* 14, no. 1 (2007): 49–53.

Ball, David J., and Sonja Boehmer-Christiansen. "Societal Concerns and Risk Decisions." *Journal of Hazardous Materials* 114 (2007): 556–63.

Ball, David, Tim Gill, and Bernard Spiegal. "Managing Risk in Play Provision: Implementation Guide." 2nd ed. London: National Children's Bureau for Play England and on behalf of Play Safety Forum, 2012. Available at http://www.playengland.org.uk/media/172644/managing-risk-in-play-provision.pdf.

Ballon, Hilary, and Kenneth T. Jackson, eds. *Robert Moses and the Modern City: The Transformation of New York*. New York: W. W. Norton, 2007.

Best, John R., Patricia H. Miller, and Lara L. Jones. "Executive Functions after Age 5: Changes and Correlates." *Developmental Review* 29 (2009): 180–200.

Blair, Clancy, and Adele Diamond. "Biological Process in Prevention and Intervention: The Promotion of Self-regulation as a Means of Preventing School Failure." *Development and Psychopathology* 20 (2008): 899–911.

Bodrova, Elena, and Deborah J. Leong. "Why Children Need Play." *Scholastic Early Childhood Today* (September 2005): 6.

———. *Tools of the Mind: The Vygotskian Approach to Early Childhood Education*. 2nd ed. Upper Saddle River, NJ: Pearson/Merrill Prentice Hall, 2007.

Bonawitz, Elizabeth, Patrick Shafto, Hyowon Gweon, Noah D. Goodman, Elizabeth Spelke, and Laura Schluz. "The Double-edged Sword of Pedagogy: Instruction Limits Spontaneous Exploration and Discovery." *Cognition* 120 (2011): 322–30.

Bonawitz, Elizabeth, Tessa J. P. van Schijndel, Daniel Friel, and Laura Schulz. "Children Balance Theories and Evidence in Exploration, Explanation, and Learning." *Cognitive Psychology* 64 (2012): 215–34.

Boyer, Ty W. "The Development of Risk-taking: A Multi-perspective Review." *Developmental Review* 26 (2006): 291–345.

Broaddus, Andrea. "Tale of Two Eco-suburbs in Freiburg, Germany: Encouraging Transit and Bicycle Use by Restricting Parking Provision." *Transportation Research Record*, no. 2187 (2010): 114–22.

Broadhead, Pat, Justine Howard, and Elizabeth Wood, eds. *Play and Learning in the Early Years: From Research to Practice*. London: Sage, 2010.

Brock, Laura, Sara E. Rimm-Kaufman, Lori Nathanson, and Kevin J. Grimm. "The Contributions of 'Hot' and 'Cold' Executive Function to Children's Academic Achievement, Learning-related Behaviours, and Engagement in Kindergarten." *Early Childhood Research* Quarterly 24 (2009): 337–49.

Brussoni, Mariana, Lise L. Olsen, Ian Pike, and David A. Sleet. "Risky Play and Children's Safety: Balancing Priorities for Optimal Child Development." *International Journal of Environmental Research and Public Health* 9, no. 9 (September 2012): 3134–48.

Bundy, Anita C., et al. "The Sydney Playground Project: Popping the Bubblewrap— Unleashing the Power of Play: A Cluster Randomized Controlled Trial of a Primary School Playground–based Intervention Aiming to Increase Children's Physical Activity and Social Skills." *BMC Public Health* 11 (2011). Available at www.biomedcetnral.com/1471-2458/11/680. Last accessed January 13, 2014.

Bundy, Anita, Tim Luckett, Paul J. Tranter, et al. "The Risk Is That There Is 'No Risk': A Simple, Innovative Intervention to Increase Children's Activity Levels." *International Journal of Early Years Education* 17, no. 1 (March 2009): 33–45.

Bunge, Silvia A., and Samantha B. Wright. "Neurodevelopmental Changes in Working Memory and Cognitive Control." *Current Opinion in Neurobiology* 17 (2007): 243–50.

Burdette, Hillary L., and Robert C. Whitaker. "A National Study of Neighborhood Safety, Outdoor Play, Television Viewing, and Obesity in Pre-school Children." *Pediatrics* 116, no. 3 (September 1, 2005): 657–62.

———. "Resurrecting Free Play in Young Children: Looking beyond Fitness and Fatness to Attention, Affiliation, and Affect." *Archives of Pediatric Adolescent Medicine* 159 (2005): 46–50.

Canning, Natalie. "The Influence of the Outdoor Environment: Den-making in Three Contexts." *European Early Childhood Education Research Journal* 8, no. 4 (2010): 555–66.

Cardon, Greet, Eveline Van Cauwenberghe, Valery Labarque, Leen Haerens, and Ilse De Bourdeaudhuij. "The Contribution of Preschool Playground Factors in Explaining Children's Physical Activity during Recess." *International Journal of Behavioral Nutrition and Physical Activity* 5, no. 11 (2008). Available at http://www.ijbnpa.org/content/5/1/11. Last accessed January 13, 2014.

Carter, Christine. *Raising Happiness: 10 Simple Steps for More Joyful Kids and Happier Parents*. New York: Ballantine Books, 2011.

Cave, Peter. *Primary School in Japan: Self, Individuality and Learning in Elementary School*. New York: Routledge, 2007.

Chaddock, Laura, Mark B. Neider, Aubrey Lutz, Charles H. Hillman, and Arthur F. Kramer. "Role of Childhood Aerobic Fitness in Successful Street Crossing." *Medicine and Science in Sports and Exercises* 44 (2012): 749–53.

Chaddock, Laura, Matthew B. Pontifex, Charles H. Hillman, and Arthur F. Kramer. "A Review of the Relation of Aerobic Fitness and Physical Activity to Brain Structure and Function in Children." *Journal of the International Neuropsychological Society* 17 (2011): 975–85.

Christakis, Dimitri, Frederick J. Zimmerman, and Michelle M. Garrison. "Effect of Block Play on Language Acquisition and Attention in Toddlers." *Archives of Pediatrics and Adolescent Medicine* 161, no. 10 (2007): 967–71.

Christiansen, Per. *Kunst ute, Kunst inne: Utsmykking Trondheim/Public Art in Trondheim 2000–2010.* Trondheim: Taour Akademisk Forlag, 2010.

Christensen, Pia, and Miguel Romero Mikkelsen. "Jumping Off and Being Careful: Children's Strategies of Risk Management in Everyday Life." *Sociology of Health and Illness* 30, no. 1 (2008): 112–30.

Claxton, Guy, and Margaret Carr. "A Framework for Teaching Learning: The Dynamics of Disposition." *Early Years: An International Research Journal* 24, no. 1 (March 2004): 87–97.

Clough, Sharyn. "Gender and the Hygiene Hypothesis." *Social Science and Medicine* 30 (2010): 1–8.

Cook, Claire, Noah D. Goodman, and Laura E. Schulz. "Where Science Starts: Spontaneous Experiments in Preschoolers' Exploratory Play." *Cognition* 1200 (2011): 341–49.

Coolahan, Kathleen, Julia Mendez, John Fantuzzo, and Paul McDermott. "Preschool Peer Interactions and Readiness to Learn: Relationships between Classroom Peer Play and Learning Behaviors and Conduct." *Journal of Educational Psychology* 92, no. 3 (September 2000): 458–65.

Cross, Gary. *Kids' Stuff: Toys and the Changing World of American Childhood.* Cambridge: Harvard University Press, 1997.

Dattner, Richard. *Design for Play.* New York: Van Nostrand Reinhold, 1969.

Davidson, Matthew C., Dima Amso, Loren Cruess Anderson, and Adele Diamond. "Development of Cognitive and Executive Functions from 4 to 13 Years: Evidence from Manipulations of Memory, Inhibition, and Task Switching." *Neuropsychologia* 44, no. 1 (2006): 2037–78.

Davis, Susan, and Nancy Eppler-Wolff. *Raising Children Who Soar: A Guide to Healthy Risk-Taking in an Uncertain World.* New York: Teachers College Press, 2009.

DeDreu, C. K., et al. "Working Memory Benefits Creative Insight, Musical Improvisation, and Original Ideation through Maintained Task-Focused Attention." *Personality and Social Psychology Bulletin* 38 (February 2, 2012): 656–69.

Diamond, Adele. "The Interplay of Biology and the Environment Broadly Defined." *Developmental Psychology* 45 (2009): 1–8.

———. "Strategies and Programs That Help to Improve Executive Functions in Young Children." Presentation at American Psychological Association, August 2009, Toronto, Canada.

———. "The Evidence Base for Improving School Outcomes by Addressing the Whole Child and by Addressing Skills and Attitudes, Not Just Content." *Early Education and Development* 21, no. 5 (September 2010): 780–93.

———. "Activities and Programs That Improve Children's Executive Functions." *Current Directions in Psychological Science* 21 (2012): 335–41.

Diamond, Adele, W. Steven Barnett, Jessica Thomas, and Sarah Munro. "Preschool Program Improves Cognitive Control." *Science* 318 (November 30, 2007): 1387–88.

Diamond, Adele, and Kathleen Lee. "Interventions Shown to Aid Executive Function Development in Children 4 to 12 Years Old." *Science* 333, no. 6045 (August 19, 2011): 959–64.

Diener, Ed, and Robert Biswas-Diener. *Happiness: Unlocking the Mysteries of Psychological Wealth.* Malden, MA: Wiley-Blackwell Publishing, 2008.

Douglas, Susan J., and Meredith W. Michaels. *The Mommy Myth: The Idealization of Motherhood and How It Has Undermined All Women*. New York: Free Press, 2005 (first published 2004).

Duckworth, Angela, Christopher Peterson, Michael Matthews, and Dennis R. Kelly. "Grit: Perseverance and Passion for Long-Term Goals." *Journal of Personality and Social Psychology* 92, no. 6 (2007): 1087–1101.

Duckworth, Angela, and Martin E. P. Seligman. "Self-Discipline Outdoes IQ in Predicting Academic Performance of Adolescents." *Psychological Science* 16 (December 2005): 939–44.

Dunn, Judy. *Children's Friendships: The Beginnings of Intimacy*. Malden, MA: Wiley-Blackwell Publishing, 2004.

Dweck, Carol. *Mindset: The New Psychology of Success*. New York: Ballantine Books, 2007.

———. "Mind Sets and Equitable Education." *Principal Leadership* 10 (January 2010): 26–29.

Eccles, Jacquelynne, and Jennifer Appleton Gootman, eds. *Community Programs to Promote Youth Development*. Washington, DC: National Academy Press, 2002.

Eigsti, Inge-Marie, Vivian Zayas, Walter Mischel, et al. "Predicting Cognitive Control from Preschool to Late Adolescence and Young Adulthood." *Psychological Science* 17, no. 6 (2006): 478–84.

Eisenberg, Nancy, Carlos Valiente, Richard A. Fabes, et al. "The Relations of Effortful Control and Ego Control to Children's Resiliency and Social Functioning." *Developmental Psychology* 39 (2003): 761–76.

Elias, Cynthia L., and Laura E. Berk. "Self-regulation in Young Children: Is There a Role for Socio-dramatic Play?" *Early Childhood Research Quarterly* 17 (2002): 216–38.

Anita C. Bundy, et al. "Increasing Physical Activity in Young Primary School Children — It's Child's Play: A Cluster Randomised Trial." *Preventive Medicine* 56 (2013): 319–25.

Eriksen, Aase. *Playground Design: Outdoor Environments for Learning and Development*. New York: Van Nostrand Reinhold Company, 1985.

Fass, Paula E., and Michael Grossberg, eds. *Reinventing Childhood after World War II*. Philadelphia: University of Pennsylvania Press, 2011.

Fischer, Claude S. *Made in America: A Social History of American Culture and Character*. Chicago: University of Chicago Press, 2010.

Fjørtoft, Ingunn. "The Natural Environment as a Playground for Children." *Early Childhood Educational Journal* 29 (Winter 2001): 111–17.

———. "Landscape as Playscape: The Effect of Natural Environments on Children's Play and Motor Development." *Children, Youth and Environments* 14, no. 2 (2004): 21–44.

Francis, Mark, and Ray Lorenzo. "Children and City Design: Proactive Process and the 'Renewal' of Childhood." In *Children and Their Environments: Learning, Using and Designing Spaces*, edited by Christopher Spencer and Mark Blades. Cambridge: Cambridge University Press, 2006.

Friedberg, M. Paul, with Ellen Perry Berkeley. *Play and Interplay: A Manifest for New Design in Urban Recreational Environment*. New York: Macmillan, 1970.

Fromberg, Doris Pronin, and Doris Bergen, eds. *Play from Birth to Twelve: Contexts, Perspectives, and Meanings*. 2nd ed. New York: Routledge, 2006.

Frost, Joe L. "The Changing Culture of Childhood: A Perfect Storm." *Childhood Education* 83, no. 4 (Summer 2007): 225–30.

Frost, Joe L., and Barry L. Klein. *Children's Play and Playgrounds*. Boston: Allyn and Bacon, 1979.

Galinsky, Ellen. *Mind in the Making: The Seven Essential Life Skills Every Child Needs*. New York: Harper Studio, 2010.

Gardner, Daniel. *The Science of Fear: How the*

Culture of Fear Manipulates Your Brain. New York: Plume, 2009 (originally published by Dutton).

Gill, Tim. *No Fear: Growing Up in a Risk Averse Society.* London: Calouste Gulbenkian Foundation, 2007.

Ginsburg, Kenneth R. "The Importance of Play in Promoting Healthy Child Development and Maintaining Strong Parent-Child Bonds." *Clinical Report from the American Academy of Pediatrics* 119 (2007): 182–91.

Ginsburg, Kenneth R., with Martha M. Jablow. *Building Resilience in Children and Teens: Giving Kids Roots and Wings.* 2nd ed. Elk Grove Village, IL: American Academy of Pediatrics, 2011.

Gopnik, Alison. *The Philosophical Baby: What Children's Minds Tell Us about Truth, Love, and the Meaning of Life.* New York: Picador, 2009.

Gopnik, Alison, Andrew N. Meltzoff, and Patricia K. Kuhl. *The Scientist in the Crib: What Early Learning Tells Us about the Mind.* New York: Harper Perennial, 2001.

Gregory, Rob, and Catherine Slessor. "Fireplace for Children." *Architectural Review* 226 (December 2009): 102–3.

Grolnick, Wendy S. *The Psychology of Parental Control: How Well-Meant Parenting Backfires.* Mahwah, NJ: Lawrence Erlbaum Associates, 2003.

———. "The Role of Parents in Facilitating Autonomous Self-regulation for Education." *Theory and Research in Education* 7, no. 2 (2009): 164–73.

Grolnick, Wendy S., and Kathy Seal. *Pressured Parents, Stressed out Kids: Dealing with Competition while Raising a Successful Child.* Amherst, NY: Prometheus Books, 2008.

Guldberg, Helene. *Reclaiming Childhood: Freedom and Play in an Age of Fear.* London: Routledge, 2009.

Harris, Paul. L. *The Work of the Imagination.* Malden MA: Blackwell Publishing, 2000.

Hart, Roger. "Containing Children: Some Lessons on Planning for Play from New York City." *Environment and Urbanization* 14 (2002): 135–48.

Healy, Jane M. *Your Child's Growing Mind.* 3rd ed. New York: Broadway Books, 2004.

Hendry, Joy. *Understanding Japanese Society.* 4th ed. New York: Routledge, 2013.

Henig, Robin Marantz. "Taking Play Seriously." *New York Times Magazine*, February 17, 2008.

Henricks, Thomas S. *Play Reconsidered: Sociological Perspectives on Human Expression.* Urbana: University of Illinois Press, 2006.

Hillman, Charles H., Kirk I. Erickson, and Arthur F. Kramer. "Be Smart, Exercise Your Heart: Exercise Effects on Brain and Cognition." *Nature* 9 (January 2008): 58–65.

Hine, Rachel, Jules Pretty, and Jo Barton. "Research Project: Social, Psychological and Cultural Benefits of Large Natural Habitat & Wilderness Experience: A Review of Current Literature for the Wilderness Foundation." Colchester: University of Essex, 2009.

Hoffman, Diane. "Risky Investments: Parenting and the Production of the 'Resilient Child.'" *Health, Risk and Society* 12 (August 2010): 385–94.

Hou, Jeffrey, ed. *Insurgent Public Space: Guerrilla Urbanism and the Remaking of Contemporary Cities.* London: Routledge, 2010.

Hughes, Fergus P. *Children, Play, and Development.* 4th ed. Los Angeles: Sage Publications, 2010.

Iacoboni, Marco. *Mirroring People: The Science of Empathy and How We Connect with Others.* New York: Picador, 2008.

Jacobs, Paul. "Playleadership Revisited." *International Journal of Early Childhood* 33, no. 2 (2001): 32–43.

Job, Veronika, Carol S. Dweck, and Gregory M. Walton. "Ego-Depletion — Is It All in Your Head? Implicit Theories about Willpower Affect Self-Regulation." *Psychological Science* 11 (2010): 1686–93.

Jones, Stephanie M., and Edward Zigler. "The

Mozart Effect: Not Learning from History." *Applied Developmental Psychology* 23 (2002): 355–72.

Kahn, Peter H., Jr. *The Human Relationship with Nature: Development and Culture.* Cambridge: MIT Press, 1999.

Kahn, Peter H., Jr., and Stephen R. Kellert, eds. *Children and Nature: Psychological, Sociocultural, and Evolutionary Investigations.* Cambridge: MIT Press, 2002.

Kamijo, Keita, Matthew B. Pontifex, Kevin C. O'Leary, Mark R. Scudder, Chien-Ting Wu, Darla M. Castelli, and Charles H. Hillman. "The Effect of an Afterschool Physical Activity Program on Working Memory in Pre-Adolescent Children." *Developmental Science* 14, no. 5 (2011): 1046–58.

Keays, G., and R. Skinner. "Playground Equipment Injuries at Home versus Those in Public Settings: Differences in Severity." *Injury Prevention* 18, no. 2 (April 2012): 38–41.

Kennison, Shelia M., and Elisabeth Ponce-Garcia. "The Role of Childhood Relationships with Older Adults in Reducing Risk-Taking by Young Adults." *Journal of Intergenerational Relationships* 10 (2012): 22–33.

Kilvington, Jacky, and Ali Wood. *Reflective Playwork.* London: Continuum International, 2010.

Kirp, David L. *Kids First: Five Big Ideas for Transforming Children's Lives and America's Future.* New York: Public Affairs, 2011.

Knight, Sara. *Risk and Adventure in Early Years Outdoor Play: Learning from Forest Schools.* London: Sage Publications, 2011.

Korpela, Kalevi, Marketta Kyttä, and Terry Hartig. "Restorative Experience, Self-regulation, and Children's Place Preferences." *Journal of Environmental Psychology* 22 (2002): 387–98.

Kuo, Frances E. "Social Aspects of Urban Forestry: The Role of Arboriculture in a Healthy Social Ecology." *Journal of Arboriculture* 29 (May 2003): 148–55.

Kuo, Frances E., and Andrea Faber Taylor. "A Potential Natural Treatment for Attention-Deficit/Hyperactivity Disorder: Evidence from a National Study." *American Journal of Public Health* 94 (September 2004): 1580–86.

Landry, Susan H., Karen E. Smith, and Paul R. Swank. "New Directions in Evaluating Social Problem Solving in Childhood: Early Precursors and Links to Adolescent Social Competence." *New Directions for Child and Adolescent Development* 123 (Spring 2009): 51–68.

Ledermann, Alfred, and Alfred Trachsel. *Creative Playgrounds and Recreation Centers.* New York: Frederick A. Praeger Publishers, 1959, 1968.

Lefaivre, Liane, and Henk Döll. *Ground-up City: Play as a Design Tool.* Translated by George Hall. Rotterdam: Nai 010 Publishers, 2007.

Lester, Stuart, and Wendy Russell. *Play England: Play for a Change: Play, Policy and Practice: A Review of Contemporary Perspectives.* London: National Children's Bureau, 2008.

Lewis, Charlie, and Jeremy I. M. Carpendale, eds. "Introduction to 'Social Interaction and the Development of Executive Function.'" Special issue of *New Direction for Child and Adolescent Development* 123 (Spring 2009).

Lindon, Jennie. *Understanding Children and Young People: Development from 5–18 Years.* London: Hodder Arnold, 2007.

Little, Helen. "Children's Risk-taking Behaviour: Implication for Early Childhood Policy and Practice." *International Journal of Early Years Education* 14 (June 2006): 141–54.

Little, Helen, and David Eager. "Risk, Challenge and Safety: Implications for Play Quality and Playground Design." *European Early Childhood Education Research Journal* 18, no. 4 (2010): 497–513.

Little, Helen, and Shirley Wyver. "Outdoor Play: Does Avoiding the Risks Reduce the Benefits?" *Australian Journal of Early Childhood* 33, no. 2 (2008): 33–40.

———. "Individual Difference in Children's Risk

Perception and Appraisals in Outdoor Play Environments." *International Journal of Early Years Education* 18, no. 4 (December 2010): 297–313.

Little, Helen, Shirley Wyver, and Frances Gibson. "The Influence of Play Context and Adult Attitudes on Young Children's Physical Risk-Taking during Outdoor Play." *European Early Childhood Education Research Journal* 19, no. 1 (2011): 113–31.

Lobo, Yovanka B., and Adam Winsler. "The Effects of a Creative Dance and Movement Program on the Social Competence of Head Start Preschoolers." *Social Development* 15 (2006): 501–19.

Lucas, Bill, and Guy Claxton. *New Kinds of Smart: How the Science of Learnable Intelligence Is Changing Education.* Maidenhead, UK: Open University Press, 2010.

Lupton, Deborah, and John Tulloch. "'Life Would Be Pretty Dull without Risk': Voluntary Risk-taking and Its Pleasures." *Health, Risk and Society* 4, no. 2 (2002): 113–24.

McGonigal, Jane. *Reality Is Broken: Why Games Make Us Better and How They Can Change the World.* New York: Penguin Group, 2011.

Medina, John. *Brain Rules for Baby: How to Raise a Smart and Happy Child from Zero to Five.* Seattle: Pear Press, 2010.

Mercogliano, Chris. *In Defense of Childhood: Protecting Kids' Inner Wildness.* Boston: Beacon Press, 2007.

Miller, Eric M., Gregory M. Walton, Carol S. Dweck, Veronika Job, Kali Trzesniewski, and Samuel M. McClure. "Theories of Willpower Affect Sustained Learning." *PLoS One* 7, no. 6 (June 2012). Available at http://www.stanford.edu/~gwalton/home/Publications_files/MillerWaltonDweckJobTrzesniewskiMcClure_2012.pdf. Last accessed January 13, 2014.

Milteer, Regina M., and Kenneth R. Ginsburg. "The Importance of Play in Promoting

Healthy Child Development and Maintaining Strong Parent-Child Bond: Focus on Children in Poverty." *Pediatrics* 129 (January 1, 2012): 204–13.

Mintz, Steven. *Huck's Raft: A History of American Childhood.* Cambridge: Belknap Press, 2004.

Mischel, Walter, Yuichi Shoda, and Philip K. Peake. "The Nature of Adolescent Competencies Predicted by Preschool Delay of Gratification." *Journal of Personality and Social Psychology* 54, no. 4 (1988): 687–96.

Moore, Robin, and Herbert H. Wong. *Natural Learning: The Life History of an Environmental School Yard.* Berkeley, CA: MIG Communications, 1997.

Moser, Thomas, and Marianne T. Martinsen. "The Outdoor Environment in Norwegian Kindergartens as Pedagogical Space for Toddlers' Play, Learning and Development." *European Early Childhood Education Research Journal* 18, no. 4 (2010): 457–71.

Moyles, Janet, ed. *The Excellence of Play.* 3rd ed. Berkshire, England: Open University Press, 2010.

Munro, Sarah, Cecil Chau, Karine Gazarian, and Adele Diamond. "Dramatically Larger Flanker Effects." Presented at the Cognitive Neuroscience Society Annual Meeting, San Francisco, CA, April 9, 2006.

Muraven, Mark, and Roy F. Baumeister. "Self-Regulation and Depletion of Limited Resources: Does Self-Control Resemble a Muscle?" *Psychological Bulletin* 126, no. 2 (2000): 247–59.

Niklasson, Laila, and Anette Sandberg. "Children and the Outdoor Environment." *European Early Childhood Education Research Journal* 18, no. 4 (2010): 485–96.

Nisbett, Richard E. *The Geography of Thought: How Asians and Westerners Think Differently . . . and Why.* New York: Free Press, 2003.

O'Brien, Liz. "Learning Outdoors: The Forest School Approach." *Education 3–13: International Journal of Primary, Elementary and Early Years Education* 37 (February 2009): 45–46.

Ogata, Amy F. "Creative Playthings: Educational Toys and Postwar American Culture." *Winterthur Portfolio* 39, nos. 2/3 (2004): 129–56.

———. *Designing the Creative Child: Playthings and Places in Midcentury America.* Minneapolis: University of Minnesota Press, 2013.

Oldenburg, Ray. *The Great Good Place.* Cambridge: Da Capo Press. 1989.

Olson, Kristina R., and Carol S. Dweck. "A Blueprint for Social Cognitive Development." *Perspectives on Psychological Science* 3 (2008): 193–202.

———. "Social Cognitive Development: A New Look." *Child Development Perspectives* 3, no. 1 (2009): 60–65.

Pellegrini, Anthony D. "Elementary School Children's Rough and Tumble Play." *Early Childhood Research Quarterly* 4 (1989): 245–60.

———. *Recess: Its Role in Education and Development.* Mahwah, NJ: Lawrence Erlbaum Associates, 2005.

———. "Research and Policy on Children's Play." *Child Development Perspectives* 3, no. 2 (2009): 131–36.

———. *The Role of Play in Human Development.* Oxford: Oxford University Press, 2009.

Pellegrini, Anthony D., and Catherine M. Bohn. "The Role of Recess in Children's Cognitive Performance and School Adjustment." *Educational Researcher* 34, no. 1 (January–February 2005): 13–19.

Pellegrini, Anthony D., Danielle Dupuis, and Peter K. Smith. "Play in Evolution and Development." *Developmental Review* 27 (2007): 261–76.

Pellis, Sergio, and Vivien Pellis. *The Playful Brain: Venturing to the Limits of Neuroscience.* Oxford: Oneworld Publications, 2009.

Pontifex, Matthew B., Mark R. Scudder, Eric S. Drollette, and Charles H. Hillman. "Fit and Vigilant: The Relationship between Poorer Aerobic Fitness and Failures in Sustained Attention during Preadolescence." *Neuropsychology* 26, no. 4 (2012): 407–13.

Putnam, Robert D., and Lewis M. Feldstein, with Don Cohen. *Better Together: Restoring the American Community.* New York: Simon and Schuster, 2003.

Reed, Peter. *Groundswell: Constructing the Contemporary Landscape.* New York: Museum of Modern Art, 2005.

Rhoades, Brittany L., Mark T. Greenberg, Stephanie T. Lanza, and Clancy Blair. "Demographic and Familial Predictors of Early Executive Function Development: Contribution of a Person-Centered Perspective." *Journal of Experimental Child Psychology* 108 (March 2011): 638–62.

Rimm-Kaufman, Sara E., Tim W. Curby, et al. "The Contribution of Children's Self-Regulation and Classroom Quality to Children's Adaptive Behaviors in the Kindergarten Classroom." *Developmental Psychology* 45 (2009): 958–72.

Robson, Sue. "Self-regulation and Metacognition in Young Children's Self-initiated Play and Reflective Dialogue." *International Journal of Early Years Education* 18, no. 3 (September 2010): 227–41.

Roseth, Cary J., Anthony D. Pellegrini, et al. "Teacher Intervention and U.S. Preschoolers' Natural Conflict Resolution after Aggressive Competition." *Behaviour* 145 (2008): 1601–26.

Ruebush, Mary. *Why Dirt Is Good: 5 Ways to Make Germs Our Friends.* New York: Kaplan Publishing, 2009.

Salovey, Peter, Marc A. Brackett, and John D. Mayer. *Emotional Intelligence: Key Reading on the Mayer and Salovey Model.* Port Chester, NY: Dude Publishing, 2004.

Sandseter, Ellen Beate Hansen. "Categorizing Risky-Play: How Can We Identify Risk-Taking in Children's Play?" *European Early Childhood Education Research Journal* 15, no. 2 (June 2007): 237–52.

———. "Affordance for Risky Play in Preschool: The Importance of Features in the Play Environment." *Early Childhood Education Journal* 36 (2009): 439–46.

———. "Characteristics of Risky Play." *Journal of Adventure Education and Outdoor Learning* 9, no. 1 (2009): 3–21.

———. "Children's Expressions of Exhilaration and Fear in Risky Play." *Contemporary Issues in Early Childhood* 10, no. 2 (2009): 92–106.

———. "'It Tickles in My Tummy!': Understanding Children's Risk-taking in Play through Reversal Theory." *Journal of Early Childhood Research* 8, no. 1 (2010): 67–88.

———. "Restrictive Safety or Unsafe Freedom? Norwegian ECEC Practitioners' Perceptions and Practices Concerning Children's Risky Play." *Child Care in Practice* 18, no. 1 (January 2012): 83–101.

Sandseter, Ellen Beate Hansen, and Leif Edward Ottesen Kennair. "Children's Risky Play from an Evolutionary Perspective: The Anti-phobic Effects of Thrilling Experiences." *Evolutionary Psychology* 9, no. 2 (2011): 257–84.

Sandseter, Ellen Beate Hansen, Helen Little, and Shirley Wyver. "Do Theory and Pedagogy Have an Impact on Provision for Outdoor Learning? A Comparison of Australia and Norway." *Journal of Adventure Education and Outdoor Learning* 12, no. 3 (2012): 167–82.

Schulz, Laura E., and Elizabeth Bonawitz. "Serious Fun: Preschoolers Engaging in More Exploratory Play when Evidence Is Confounded." *Developmental Psychology* 43, no. 4 (2007): 1045–50.

Schulz, Laura, Holly R. Standing, and Elizabeth B. Bonawitz. "Word, Thought, and Deed: The Role of Object Categories in Children's Inductive Inferences and Exploratory Play." *Developmental Psychology* 44, no. 5 (2008): 1266–76.

Seligman, Martin E. P. *Flourish*. New York: Free Press, 2011.

Seymour, Whitney North, Jr., ed. *Small Urban Spaces: The Philosophy, Design, Sociology, and Politics of Vest-pocket Parks and Other Small Urban Open Spaces*. New York: New York University Press, 1969.

Shaw, Ben, Ben Watson, Bjorn Frauendienst, Andreas Redecker, Tim Jones, and Mayer Hillman. "Children's Independent Mobility: A Comparative Study in England and Germany (1971–2010)." Policy Studies Institute. Available at http://www.psi.org.uk/site/publication_detail/852. Last accessed January 13, 2014.

Shin, Huiyoung, and Allison M. Ryan. "How Do Adolescents Cope with Social Problems?: An Examination of Social Goals, Coping with Friends, and Social Adjustment." *Journal of Early Adolescence* 32, no. 6 (2012): 851–75.

Shonkoff, Jack P., and Deborah A. Phillips, eds. *From Neurons to Neighborhoods: The Science of Early Childhood Development*. Washington, DC: National Academy Press, 2000.

Shooter, Mike, and Sue Baily, eds. *The Young Mind*. London: Bantam and the Royal College of Psychiatrists, 2009.

Singer, Dorothy G., Roberta M. Golinkoff, and Kathy Hirsh-Pasek, eds. *Play=Learning: How Play Motivates and Enhances Children's Cognitive and Social-Emotional Growth*. New York: Oxford University Press, 2006.

Smith, Peter K. *Children and Play*. Malden, MA: Wiley-Blackwell, 2010.

Smith, Peter K., and Craig H. Hart, eds. *Blackwell Handbook of Childhood Social Development*. Malden, MA: Wiley-Blackwell, 2004.

Solomon, Susan G. *American Playgrounds: Revitalizing Community Space*. Hanover and London: 2005.

———. "Artful Playscapes." *Public Art Review* (Fall/Winter 2011): 48–53.

Staempfli, Marianne B. "Reintroducing Adventure into Children's Outdoor Play Environments." *Environment and Behavior* 41 (2009): 268–80.

Stipek, Deborah, Stephen Newton, and Amita Chudgar. "Learning-related Behaviors and Literacy Achievement in Elementary School–aged Children." *Early Childhood Research Quarterly* 25 (2010): 385–95.

Storli, Rune, and Trond Løge Hagen. "Affordances in Outdoor Environments and Children's Physically Active Play in Pre-School." *European Early Childhood Education Research Journal* 18, no. 4 (2010): 445–56.

Taylor, Andrea Faber, and Frances E. Kuo. "Is Contact with Nature Important for Healthy Child Development?: State of the Evidence." In *Children and Their Environments: Learning, Using and Designing Spaces*, edited by Christopher Spencer and Mark Blades. Cambridge: Cambridge University Press, 2006.

———. "Children with Attention Deficits Concentrate Better after Walk in the Park." *Journal of Attention Disorders* 12 (2009): 402–9.

———. "Could Exposure to Everyday Green Spaces Help Treat ADHD? Evidence from Children's Play Settings." *Applied Psychology: Health and Well-Being* 3 (2011): 281–303.

Taylor, Andrea Faber, Frances E. Kuo, and William C. Sullivan. "Copying with ADD: The Surprising Connection to Green Play Settings." *Environment and Behaviour* 33 (2001): 54–75.

———. "Views of Nature and Self-Discipline: Evidence from Inner City Children." *Journal of Environmental Psychology* 22 (2002): 49–63.

Thom, Betsy, Rosemary Sales, and Jenny J. Pearce, eds. *Growing Up with Risk*. Bristol: Policy Press, 2007.

Tobin, Joseph, Yeh Hsueh, and Mayumi Karasawa. *Preschool in Three Cultures Revisited: China, Japan, and the United States*. Chicago: University of Chicago Press, 2009.

Tough, Paul. *How Children Succeed: Grit, Curiosity, and the Hidden Power of Character*. Boston: Houghton Mifflin Harcourt, 2012.

Tovey, Helen. *Playing Outdoors: Spaces and Places, Risk and Challenge*. New York: McGraw Hill, 2007.

Trainor, James. "Reimagining Recreation." *Cabinet* 45 (Spring 2012). Available at http://cabinetmagazine.org/issues/45/trainor.php. Last accessed January 13, 2014.

Vollman, David, Rachel Witsaman, et al. "Epidemiology of Playground Equipment-Related Injuries to Children in the United States, 1996–2005." *Clinical Pediatrics* 48 (January 2009): 66–71.

Waldfogel, Jane. *What Children Need*. Cambridge: Harvard University Press, 2006.

Waller, Tim, Ellen Beate H. Sandseter, Shirley Wyver, Eva Ärlemalm-Hagser, and Trisha Maynard. "The Dynamics of Early Childhood Spaces: Opportunities for Outdoor Play?" *European Early Childhood Education Research Journal* 18, no. 4 (2010): 437–43.

Warner, Judith. *Perfect Madness: Motherhood in the Age of Anxiety*. New York: Riverhead Books, 2005.

Waters, Jane, and Sharon Begley. "Supporting the Development of Risk Taking Behaviours in the Early Years: An Exploratory Study." *International Journal of Primary, Elementary and Early Years Education* 35, no. 4 (May 2008): 365–77.

Waters, Jane, and Trisha Maynard. "What Is So Interesting Outside? A Study of Child-Initiated Interaction with Teachers in the Natural Outdoor Environment." *European Early Childhood Education Research Journal* 18, no. 4 (2010): 473–83.

Willoughby, M. T., R. J. Wirth, C. B. Blair, and Family Life Project Investigators. "Executive Function in Early Childhood: Longitudinal Measurement Invariance and Developmental Change." *Psychological Assessment* 24, no. 2 (October 24, 2011): 418–431.

Wyver, Shirley R., and Susan H. Spence. "Play and Divergent Problem-Solving: Evidence Supporting a Reciprocal Relationship."

Early Education and Development 10, no. 4 (October 1999).

Wyver, Shirley, Paul Tranter, Geraldine Naughton, Helen Little, Ellen Beate Hansen Sandseter, and Anita Bundy. "Ten Ways to Restrict Children's Freedom to Play: The Problem of Surplus Safety." *Contemporary Issues in Early Childhood* 11, no. 3 (2010). Available at www.wwwords.co.uk/CIEC. Last accessed January 13, 2014.

Index

Page numbers in *italics* refer to illustrations.